Nourishing
THE FIGHTER

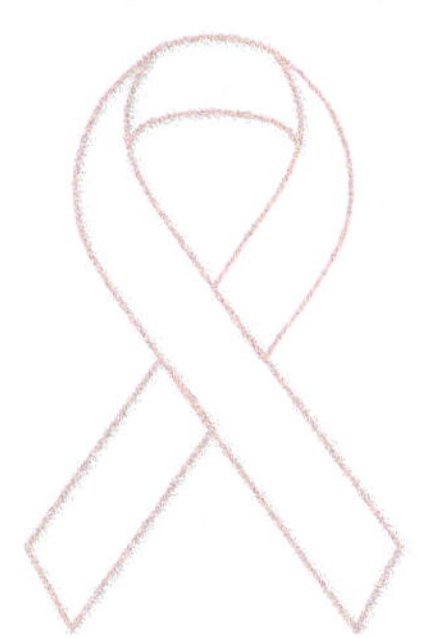

LEILA DAVIES-FRICK

Design **Collette Sadler**
Editor **Garima Sharma**
Photography **Jodielee Photography**

Image credits
p4 author's own photograph
p64, 71, 83, 87, 91, 95 Jodielee Photography
*p20, 21, 22, 24, 25, 26, 27, 28, 29, 32, 33,
34, 36, 37, 38, 39, 40, 41, 67, 72, 88* used with
permission from Unsplash.

p35, 78, 92 used with permission
from Freepick.

ACKNOWLEDGEMENTS
Leila Davies-Frick acknowledges the
Traditional Custodians of the country
throughout Australia and their connection
to lands, water and communities. We pay
out respect to elders past and present and
respect to all Aboriginal and Torres Strait
Islander people today.

AUTHOR'S ACCREDITATIONS
Diploma in Child Studies; TAFE SA
Certificate: Nutrition, Children's Nutrition,
and Nutrition for Disease Management;
Health Academy Australia

I write this book to give hope and strength to parents and caregivers, when all seems lost and out of your hands. I hope that my own experience provides you with relevant information to lessen the impact of cancer treatment on your children.

In memory of Tyrone and Liam, thank you for the laughter and smiles you brought to myself and Jake.

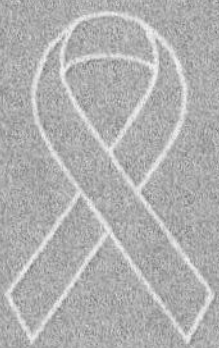

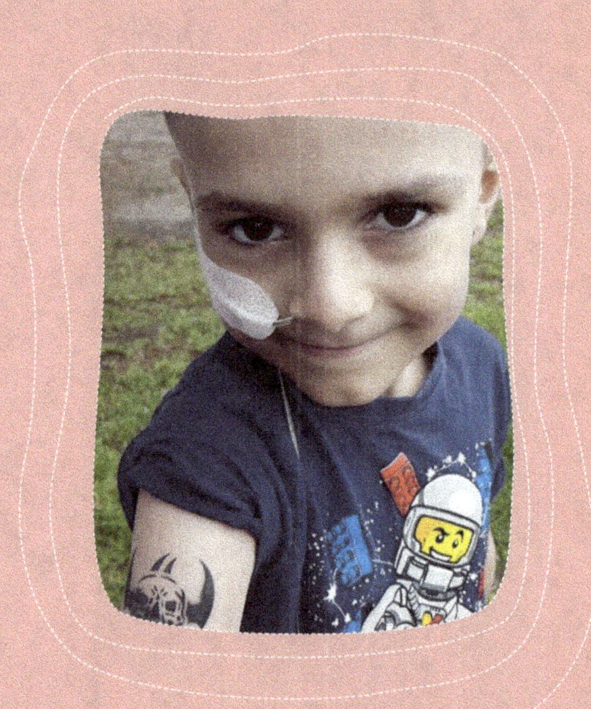

Your battle is my battle ❤ Mum

CONTENTS

INTRODUCTION

INTRODUCTION

As I sit here, donating plasma at the lifeblood centre, my mind wanders back to the reason why I started this journey in the first place. The date remains etched in my heart forever. It was 16 April 2015 when life dealt us a heavy blow – the day we received the devastating news, "Yep, it's Cancer." It was conveyed to us in such a blunt manner, leaving us stunned and in disbelief.

Just a short while before, we had been on Easter holidays, and my son Jake (6 years old) seemed a bit off, but still, he played with his cousins and rode his bike. On that fateful day, we had planned to go to shops and get supplies to bake cakes. Jake asked to ride in his baby sister's pram because he was feeling tired. In retrospect, I see that moment as a crossroad – I could have simply taken him home to rest, attributing his fatigue to the busy weekend we had. However, something instinctive led me to choose the hospital instead. With three young children in tow, we rushed to Noarlunga Hospital. I do not recall how long we waited, but I vividly remember the events that followed once we reached the emergency department.

The doctor examined Jake, and I mentioned that he had been unusually tired and complained of a sore stomach. All relevant blood tests were conducted, and while we waited for the results, the doctor checked his vitals, listened to his breathing, and performed a tap test on his stomach, making Jake giggle. The doctor assured us that everything seemed fine and suspected a stomach virus that was going around at the time, but as a precaution, he wanted to do a chest X-ray owing to Jake's history of asthma. Jake experienced multiple hospitalisation visits due to asthma attacks, which began when he was just a few months old. As the X-ray results were alarming, the doctor ordered an ultrasound to investigate further. Panic began to set in when the sonographer called in their boss to look. The truth hit us like a ton of bricks when the man confirmed, in front of Jake, that he had cancer. We were in shock, and the doctor apologized, assuming we had already been informed.

Just hit by a curveball, life took an overwhelming turn from that moment. We rushed to Women's and Children's Hospital in North Adelaide, leaving my daughters behind as we prepared for the challenging road ahead. After multiple tests and biopsies, we received the heartbreaking diagnosis the following day: Jake had Stage 4 Neuroblastoma, affecting various areas including his throat, chest, stomach, and spine.

What followed were gruelling rounds of chemotherapy, surgeries, radiotherapy, and cell transplants, along with numerous complications and weight loss. As parents, we were now faced with the difficult task of saying "yes" to treatments that caused our child pain and suffering. Watching our son turn frail while enduring all this was heart-wrenching. In my desire to find some semblance of control, I focused on Jake's nutrition during his treatment. I connected with Jake's nutritionist at WCH, and expressed my concerns. Together, we worked to improve the ward menu, incorporating healthier options and a rotating schedule to avoid monotony. Besides, we ensured that children could order comfort foods, such as nuggets and chips, on call. Despite the incredible support we received from the medical team, I could not help but feel that more could be done regarding nutrition and overall well-being during treatment. This thought sparked the idea of sharing our journey, along with tips and tricks that helped us navigate through treatment and its aftermath.

Through this book, I hope to offer support and guidance to others facing similar challenges, to let them know they are not alone on this arduous journey. Let us walk together with hope and determination. xx

THE INTRICATE DANCE OF TREATMENT:
UNVEILING THE IMPACT ON DIET AND HEALTH

It is a catch-22 situation, I believe. On one hand, we need treatment to combat and eliminate cancer cells; on the other hand, it affects patients' healthy cells, tissues, and organs. We can only hope that patients' bodies are resilient enough to handle the treatment's impact and continue fighting.

Amidst a wide array of adverse effects that cancer treatment has on human body, one significant side effect is malnutrition, which stems from various factors like changes in taste, smell, appetite, and the body's ability to eat sufficient food or absorb essential nutrients needed for a healthy functioning body.

Given below are some of the common treatments that paediatric cases may undergo and the potential effects they might cause:

CHEMOTHERAPY	SURGERY
Irritation of mouth lining leading to stomatitis at times	Inability to eat or reduced appetite
Sore mouth and inflammation	Fatigue
Irritation of the digestive tract	Altered taste perception
Altered taste perception	Difficulty in eating (eating difficulties may vary depending on the location of surgery)
Increased susceptibility to infections	Periods of digestive system dysfunction
Fatigue	
Diarrhoea	
Nausea and vomiting	
Decreased red blood cells/haemoglobin causing anaemia	

RADIOTHERAPY	STEM CELL AND BONE MARROW TRANSPLANTS
Inflammation around the treatment site	Mouth and throat pain
Reduced appetite	Nausea and vomiting
Fatigue	Weakened immune system
Nausea or sickness	Fatigue
Sore mouth	Low platelet count, leading to difficulty in blood clotting
Diarrhoea	Diarrhoea
	Low red blood cell count

Besides the direct treatment effects, other factors can also influence your child's eating habits during treatment, such as the hospital environment, depression, pain, and changes in taste and smell. Not to mention, DNA damage can also occur as a side effect of conventional cancer treatments like chemotherapy and radiotherapy. While these treatments are effective in killing cancer cells, they can also harm healthy cells and their DNA. Unfortunately, this damage may increase the risk of developing secondary cancers in patients who have successfully completed their cancer treatment. Hence, it is crucial to be aware of the potential toll that treatments can take on your child's health. To support their well-being, it can be beneficial to incorporate foods into their diet that possess DNA-protecting properties. Based on the latest research, some foods rich in nucleic acids, such as meat, fish, seafood, legumes, and mushrooms, can help boost children's defences and protect their DNA. Hence, incorporating these foods items in your child's diet can provide valuable nutrients and support their overall health.

Despite our immense luck with Jake responding well to all his treatments, it was not without enduring significant pain. Jake encountered various side effects, ranging in severity, during most of his treatments and battles with colds. Many of his treatments involved blood and plasma donations. As the treatment progressed, fatigue became a major issue, eventually requiring the use of a wheelchair for mobility outside the house. Unfortunately, the first chemotherapy treatment brought about hair loss and a loss of appetite, leading to rapid weight loss. Moreover, some treatments and surgeries resulted in ICU stays.

Throughout our journey, I will share how we did our best to manage these challenges and offer insights to help you cope.

THE IMPACT OF PSYCHOLOGICAL FACTORS ON NUTRITION DURING TREATMENT

It is not just chemotherapy and radiotherapy that will affect your child's food intake. Several other factors come into play. Given below are some of these:

HOSPITAL ENVIRONMENT: After Jake's first stay, he knew what to expect and how he would feel, which triggered his anxiety. Whenever I had control over the environment, I made sure to create a fun atmosphere and turned mealtime into special moments. During lunchtime, we used to have our special "lunch date." Jake would often sleep most of the morning, but miraculously wake up just in time for us to share a meal and enjoy watching Ellen together. It was precious quality time, and the humour from the show would distract him, making him more likely to eat. Jake also had a keen interest in the cooking channel, especially shows hosted by Curtis Stone, Jamie Oliver, and MasterChef. Watching these culinary delights not only increased his appetite but also inspired me to up my game in the kitchen.

DEPRESSION: The emotional impact of the treatment journey can lead to a loss of appetite, reduced appetite, or complete disinterest in food. Moreover, the changing appearance due to treatment could further contribute to depression depending on your child age.

PAIN WHEN EATING: Some treatments can cause discomfort or pain while eating, making it all the more challenging to consume an adequate amount of food.

NAUSEA, VOMITING, AND DIARRHOEA: Despite using helpful aids like wafers, there are days during and after treatment when even those measures may not provide relief. Identifying triggers and preventing them can be beneficial. For instance, if certain foods consistently induce vomiting, it is best to avoid them. Over time, even the thought of those foods may become unappealing. Jake developed two main triggers: chocolate cake and hot chips. As a result, we had to be cautious about his food choices. Even at the hospital, we had to leave Jake's food outside of his room because the container used to keep it warm became an additional trigger.

In addition, we found that changing to odourless cleaning products or those without strong smells and allowing food to air out before bringing it into the room helped. In hospitals, requesting alternative cleaning products or having food left outside the room can be options worth exploring.

While we cannot eliminate these side effects, we can take steps to minimise their impact. Some tips we found useful were:

- serving room temperature meals
- avoiding fluids while eating
- engaging in mild physical activities or getting fresh air when the child feels up to it
- sitting upright while eating and for an hour afterward, if possible

CHANGE IN TASTE/TASTE BUDS: Approximately 50% of those undergoing treatment experience changes in taste; these alterations can occur shortly after treatment or gradually over the next few days. Some of the taste changes include bitterness, metallic taste, excessive sweetness, or loss of taste altogether. Taste buds typically recover within 1 to 2 months after treatment.

Tips to overcome taste changes include:

- avoid eating 2-3 hours after treatment;
- mask the metallic taste with lemonade (except when experiencing dry mouth or mouth sores);
- use plastic utensils;
- use strong herbs when cooking;
- marinate foods with flavourful sauces like tomato or BBQ; and
- freshen the palate between meals with minty toothpaste or mints.

SMELLS: Smells can have a significant impact on appetite, especially if they trigger negative associations. For Jake, certain smells related to foods he had eaten and then vomited would cause nausea. Also, cleaning products were a source of discomfort. We had to eliminate or change a variety of things as his treatment progressed.

Food-related strategies to manage smells include opting for mild foods with minimal odour, such as custards, mousse, yogurt, dry biscuits, crackers, and noodles. Although these mild foods may not be particularly appetizing, they can provide something to fill their bellies.

MOUTH SORES/DRY MOUTH: This condition can make eating difficult and uncomfortable. Some relief measures include:

- consuming soft foods;
- cutting food into small pieces;
- opting for cold foods;
- using sauces and gravies to aid in swallowing;
- avoiding citrus, spicy, and salty foods;
- using fragrance-free lip balm;
- sucking on lollies or candies;
- having ice and icy poles (if allowed during treatment);
- taking small sips of water, using a spoon if lips are too sore for a straw; or
- choosing water-rich foods, such as cucumbers and watermelons, which are gentle, cooling, and hydrating.

By understanding and addressing these factors, we can work towards ensuring our children receive adequate nutrition during their treatment journey.

BUILDING STRENGTH FROM WITHIN: THE POWERFUL IMPACT OF NUTRITIONAL SUPPORT

Cancer and its treatments can greatly impact your child's eating habits and how well they tolerate food. Hence, it becomes all the more important to provide their bodies with a diverse range of nutritious foods ant, thus, fulfill its nutritional needs. Given below are some key benefits of maintaining a healthy diet:

LOWERING BLOOD PRESSURE: A healthy diet can decrease high blood pressure levels, promote cardiovascular health, and attain overall well-being. (This can help when taking certain medication.)

DECREASING HIGH CHOLESTEROL LEVELS: Adopting a nutritious eating plan can enable actively working towards lowering cholesterol levels and improving heart health.

ENHANCING YOUR STATE OF HEALTH: Good nutrition plays a vital role in supporting your overall health, providing essential nutrients for the body to function optimally.

STRENGTHENING YOUR IMMUNE SYSTEM: A balanced diet boosts your immune system, increasing body's resistance to diseases and infections.

Besides these benefits, adhering to a healthy diet during cancer treatment offers several advantages:

FEELING BETTER: Proper nutrition can contribute to a sense of well-being and improved energy levels, enabling you to cope better with the challenges of treatment.

FASTER HEALING: A well-nourished body has a greater capacity to heal and recover from the side effects of cancer treatments.

SUPPORTING GROWTH AND DEVELOPMENT: Adequate nutrition is paramount for children and adolescents undergoing cancer treatment, for it aids in healthy growth and development.

IMPROVING QUALITY OF LIFE: Good nutrition can enhance the overall quality of life by reducing treatment-related symptoms and increasing your ability to perform activities of daily life.

Moreover, following a healthy diet can lower the risk of infections. Throughout your diagnosis, treatment, and beyond, you may experience changes in appetite, diet, and nutritional status due to treatment side effects or disease symptoms. Symptoms like dry mouth, altered taste and appetite, nausea, diarrhoea, and vomiting can lead to poor nutrient intake and absorption. Hence, prioritising good nutrition in this scenario can decrease the likelihood of infections and support your body's ability to fight off illnesses. Furthermore, recognising the importance of maintaining a healthy diet can enable you to optimise overall well-being and improve your ability to navigate the challenges of cancer and its treatments.

Cancer can also cause weight loss and malnutrition in patients. When someone has cancer, their body may lose muscle and weight, medically known as cachexia – a condition that can make patients very weak. This happens because of the body's response to the tumour, changes in metabolism, and how the body uses nutrients. Poor nutrition is common among cancer patients and can make their overall well-being worse and affect how well their treatment works. A plethora of medical evidence establishes a correlation between cancer and poor nutrition. Thus, having poor nutrition while undergoing cancer treatment can make things more difficult. It weakens the immune system, making it easier to get infections and have complications during treatment. Furthermore, poor nutrition can make treatment less effective and cause delays, making it even harder for the body to fight cancer cells.

A study published in the Journal of Clinical Oncology demonstrated that cancer patients who were well-nourished did better with chemotherapy, had fewer side effects, and responded better to treatment compared with malnourished patients. Over the years, many studies have established that getting the right nutrition at the right time can help patients tolerate treatment better, have fewer side effects, and possibly achieve better results. Therefore, not getting sufficient nutrition can also make people feel physically and mentally worse. Malnourished cancer patients often feel tired, weak, and have difficulty doing everyday activities. Besides, they may experience sadness or anxiety, further making it harder for them to follow their treatment plan and feel emotionally well. To address these problems, it's essential for doctors, dietitians, and other healthcare professionals to work together. They can provide support such as counselling, nutritional supplements, and sometimes even feeding tubes or intravenous nutrition. Hence, it is crucial to address malnutrition with proper support to improve patients' response to treatment, their overall well-being, and their chances of recovery.

REFERENCE:

Na BG, Han SS, Cho YA, Wie GA, Kim JY, Lee JM, Lee SD, Kim SH, Park SJ. Nutritional Status of Patients with Cancer: A Prospective Cohort Study of 1,588 Hospitalized Patients. Nutr Cancer. 2018 Nov-Dec;70(8):1228-1236. doi: 10.1080/01635581.2019.1578392. Epub 2019 Mar 22. PMID: 30900926.

NATURE'S BOUNTY

This chapter explores a variety of colourful and healthy foods that are packed with nutrients to strengthen our body's defences against illnesses. From juicy fruits to wholesome vegetables, these immune-boosting options can be a great addition to your child's diet, especially during chemotherapy and stem cell therapy.

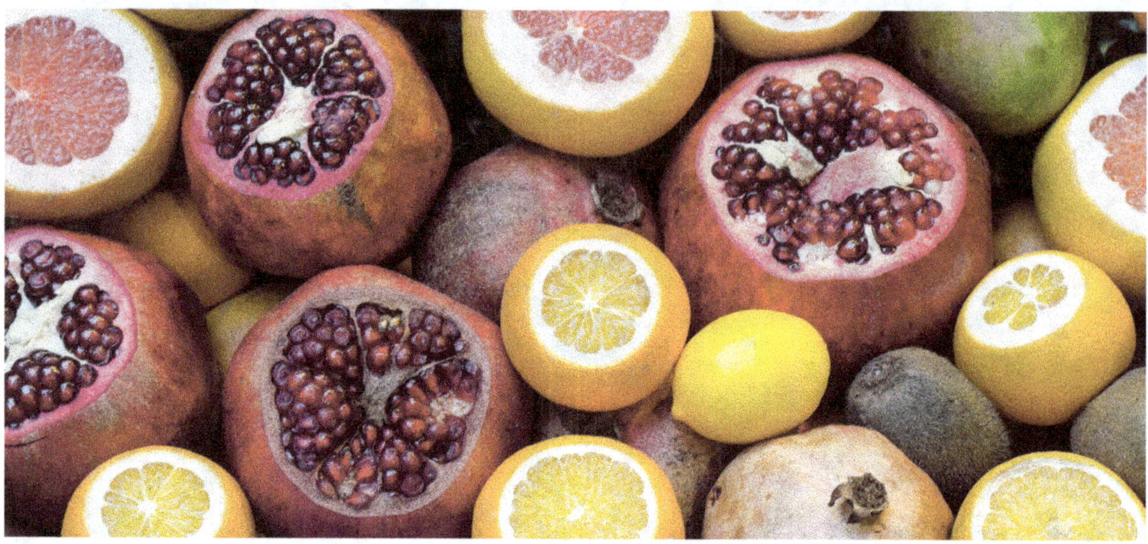

POWER OF IMMUNE-ACTIVATING FOODS Foods like blackberries, walnuts, and pomegranates play a vital role in activating your child's immune system. As our immune system works hard to protect our health, adding these nutrient-rich delights to your child's meals can be beneficial, especially during medical treatment.

STRENGTHENING YOUR BODY'S DEFENCES: Keeping the immune system strong is vital, especially during advanced cancer immunotherapies that rely on a robust immune response for the best results. By enjoying an assortment of immune-boosting foods, you provide your child's body with what it needs to keep its protective shield at its best.

Through the wonders of nature's bounty, we will explore a palette of foods that not only taste great but also offer plentiful health benefits. With these immune-boosting nutrition tips, you can take care of your child's well-being and support their immune system throughout their cancer treatment journey.

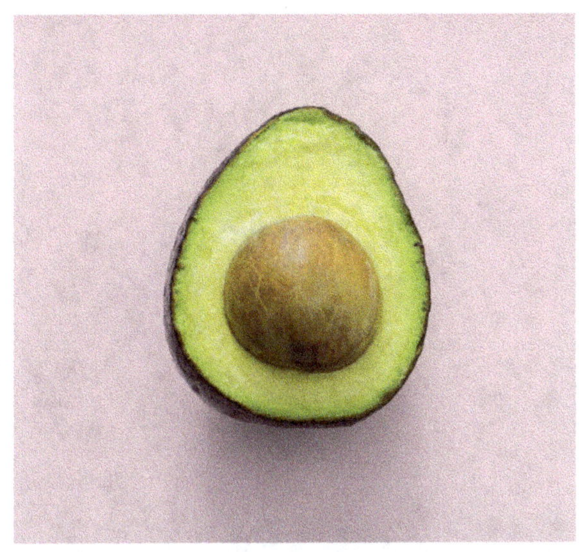

FRUITS

AVOCADOS

Avocados (Persea americana), with proven anti-carcinogenic properties, are renowned for providing abundant health benefits, primarily because of their high monounsaturated fat content – a type of fat that is beneficial for overall health, especially in terms of cardiovascular health, as it helps in lowering cholesterol levels. In fact, magnesium in avocados supports a healthy heart. In addition, avocados provide valuable nutrients like vitamin E, vitamin C, vitamin K, potassium, and fibre, further boosting the immune system. The presence of lutein helps in avoiding eye cataracts and macular degeneration. With such a diverse range of advantages, including avocados in our diet can contribute to a well-rounded and nourishing approach to overall wellness.

References:

Dreher ML, Davenport AJ. Hass avocado composition and potential health effects. Crit Rev Food Sci Nutr. 2013;53(7):738-50. doi: 10.1080/10408398.2011.556759. PMID:23638933; PMCID: PMC3664913.

Dabas D, Elias RJ, Ziegler GR, et al. In Vitro Antioxidant and Cancer Inhibitory Activity of a Colored Avocado Seed Extract. Int J Food Sci. 2019 Apr 24;2019:6509421. doi: 10.1155/2019/6509421. PMID: 31179313; PMCID: PMC6507236.

Galván GC, Freedland SJ. Avocados: a recipe for good guacamole or lower cancer risk? Cancer Prev Res (Phila). 2023 Apr 3;16(4):187-189. doi: 10.1158/1940-6207.CAPR-23-0031. PMID: 37009710.

GRAPES

Grapes (genus Vitis) are a treasure trove of health-enhancing polyphenols, such as anthocyanins, flavanols, flavonols, and resveratrol, making them a valuable addition to any diet. These polyphenols have been linked to various health benefits owing to their antioxidant, cardioprotective, anticancer, anti-inflammation, antiaging, and antimicrobial properties, thereby significantly affecting cardiovascular health and even preventing cancer. From the class of flavonols, quercetin is a phenolic compound that exhibits anti-clotting properties, aiding in maintaining a healthy circulatory system. Grapes also boast antiviral and antifungal properties, contributing to their ability to support the body's immune defences. Moreover, they serve as an excellent source of vitamin C, an essential nutrient for maintaining a strong immune system and overall well-being. Hence, embracing the natural goodness of grapes in our daily nutrition can be a simple yet effective way to boost our health and wellness.

References:

Zhou K, Raffoul JJ. Potential anticancer properties of grape antioxidants. J Oncol. 2012;2012:803294. doi: 10.1155/2012/803294. Epub 2012 Aug 7. PMID: 22919383; PMCID: PMC3420094.

Kaur M, Agarwal C, Agarwal R. Anticancer and cancer chemopreventive potential of grape seed extract and other grape-based products. J Nutr. 2009 Sep;139(9):1806S-12S. doi: 10.3945/jn.109.106864. Epub 2009 Jul 29. PMID: 19640973; PMCID: PMC2728696.

FIGS

Figs (genus Ficus) offer a delightful blend of taste and health benefits, making them a wholesome addition to our diet. Besides offering a myriad of health benefits, figs have been proven to contain a potent anticancer agent. Rich in natural energy and sugars, these succulent fruits provide a quick and nourishing pick-me-up, ideal for refuelling during busy days. In addition, figs are a valuable source of potassium, which help in maintaining proper fluid balance and preventing unwanted fluid retention. When opting for dried figs, we reap the rewards of increased iron content, which contributes to improved blood quality and boosts calcium levels, supporting healthy bones. When out of season, Fig Vinegar can also be considered, as it is a robust detoxifier. Besides, incorporating Fig Vinegar to diet plans can help reap the benefits of its anti-inflammatory, antioxidant, and anticancer properties. Hence, embracing the goodness of figs in our daily routine can be a tasty and nutritious way to enhance our overall well-being.

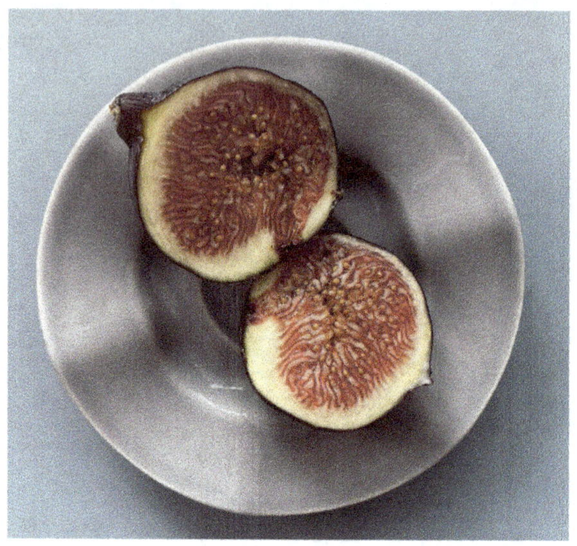

References:

Lightbourn AV, Thomas RD. Crude edible fig (Ficus carica) leaf extract prevents diethylstilbestrol (DES)-induced DNA strand breaks in single-cell gel electrophoresis (SCGE)/comet assay: literature review and pilot study. J Bioequivalence Bioavailab. 2019;11(2):19-28. doi: 10.35248/0975-0851.19.11.389. Epub 2019 Apr 1. PMID: 31814674; PMCID: PMC6897490.

Rasool IFU, Aziz A, Khalid W, et al. Industrial application and health prospective of fig (Ficus carica) by-products. Molecules. 2023 Jan 18;28(3):960. doi: 10.3390/molecules 28030960. PMID: 36770628; PMCID: PMC 9919570.

MANGOES

Mangoes (genus Mangifera), often hailed as nutrient superheroes, bring an array of health benefits to the table. One of their standout attributes is being a valuable source of vitamin C, a potent immune-boosting vitamin that supports our body's defence system. With high potassium content, mangoes contribute to the regulation of blood sugar levels and promoting overall cardiovascular health. Another key component in mangoes is pectin, a high level of soluble fibre that aids in digestion and supports a healthy gut. Beyond these remarkable qualities, mangoes are a nutrient powerhouse, providing us with a wealth of other essential nutrients that contribute to our well-being. In addition, mangoes contain an anticancer compound called mangiferin, which helps in reducing inflammation and boosts the immune system. Per the latest research, mango extracts have been shown to inhibit the spread of cancer cells and even decrease the size of cancerous tumours, particularly breast cancer. Hence, including mangoes in our diet can be a delightful way to bolster our health and relish the tropical flavours they offer.

References:

Deng Q, Tian YX, Liang J. Mangiferin inhibits cell migration and invasion through Rac1/ WAVE2 signalling in breast cancer. Cytotechnology. 2018 Apr;70(2):593-601. doi: 10.1007/s10616-017-0140-1. Epub 2018 Feb 17. PMID: 29455393; PMCID: PMC5851954.

Du M, Wen G, Jin J, Chen Y, Cao J, Xu A. Mangiferin prevents the growth of gastric carcinoma by blocking the PI3K-Akt signalling pathway. Anticancer Drugs. 2018 Feb; 29(2):167-175. doi: 10.1097/CAD. 00000000 00000583. PMID: 29215373.

PEARS

Pears (genus Pyrus), with their high fibre content and antioxidant properties, make a delightful and healthful addition to our diet. One of the remarkable qualities of pears is their allergy-friendly nature, rendering them largely safe for individuals with allergies. Beyond that, pears are packed with an array of essential nutrients, making them a nutrient-rich choice for promoting overall well-being. In addition, pears (mainly the core) contain hydroxycinnamic acids, which act as potent antioxidants with potential anticancer and antibacterial properties, further bolstering their health benefits. In contrast, the pear peel has abundant anthocyanins, flavonols, catechins, and procyanidins, along with high levels of antioxidants, including vitamin C, vitamin K, and copper. In particular, copper in pears is known to boost body's immune system, which is beneficial in cancer treatment. In fact, pears are expected to contain further cancer-fighting compounds, although this is still under investigation. In the meanwhile, enjoying pears as a regular part of our diet can be a delicious way to support our health and savour the goodness they have to offer.

References:

Reiland H, Slavin J. Systematic review of pears and health. Nutr Today. 2015 Nov;50(6):301-305. doi: 10.1097/NT.000000 0000000112. Epub 2015 Nov 23. PMID: 26663955; PMCID: PMC4657810.

Hong SY, Lansky E, Kang SS, et al. A review of pears (Pyrus spp.), ancient functional food for modern times. BMC Complement Med Ther. 2021 Sep 1;21(1):219. doi: 10.1186/s12906-021-03392-1. PMID: 34470625; PMCID: PMC 8409479.

Ajmera R. Fruits to eat during and after cancer treatment. Healthline. August 28, 2019. Available at https://www.healthline. com/nutrition/fruits-for-cancer-patients

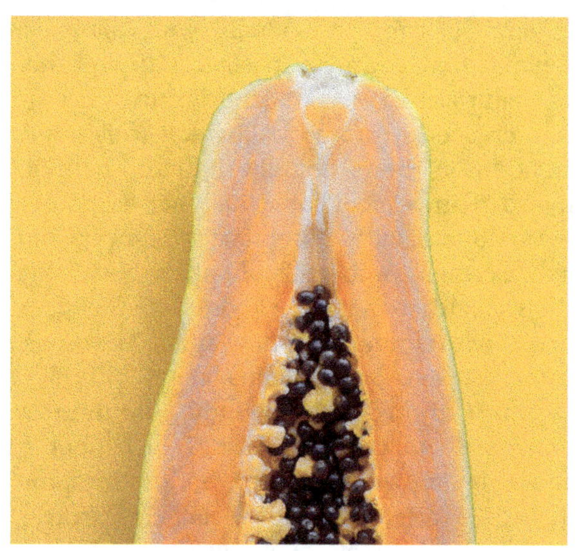

PAPAYAS

Papayas (genus Carica), a tropical fruit, are truly a nutritional powerhouse, brimming with essential nutrients that support our health manifold. One of the standout components in papayas is beta-carotene, a valuable compound that our body converts into vitamin A, promoting excellent vision and overall well-being. Another noteworthy nutrient is beta-cryptoxanthin, which supports lung health and may contribute to a well-functioning respiratory system. Moreover, lutein and zeaxanthin in papayas are antioxidants that are essential in protecting our eyes from macular degeneration, helping maintain healthy vision. Besides these carotenes, papayas boast a rich content of vitamin C and dietary fibre, both beneficial for our immune system and digestive health, respectively. The abundance of vitamin C helps fortify our immune defences, aiding in warding off illnesses and keeping us healthy. The fibre in papayas supports smooth digestion and helps maintain bowel regularity, contributing to overall digestive wellness. Furthermore, papayas have been linked to blood sugar regulation, as they possess natural compounds that could slow the rise of blood sugar levels, rendering them particularly beneficial for individuals managing their blood sugar levels or those at risk of developing diabetes. Indeed, a number of studies have demonstrated that the papaya fruit, seeds, or leaves extracts possess cytotoxic and antiproliferative activities for numerous cancer types like breast cancer, liver cancer, cervical cancer, lung cancer, and pancreatic cancer. Therefore, incorporating papayas into our diet can be a delightful and healthful choice. Enjoying the delicious taste of papayas while reaping their impressive health benefits is a win-win for our overall health and happiness.

References:

Schweiggert RM, Kopec RE, Villalobos-Gutierrez MG, et al. Carotenoids are more bioavailable from papaya than from tomato and carrot in humans: a randomised cross-over study. Br J Nutr. 2014 Feb;111(3):490-8. doi: 10.1017/S0007114513002596. Epub 2013 Aug 12. PMID: 23931131; PMCID: PMC4091614.

Pandey S, Cabot PJ, Shaw PN, et al. Anti-inflammatory and immunomodulatory properties of Carica papaya. J Immunotoxicol. 2016 Jul;13(4):590-602. doi: 10.3109/1547691X.2016.1149528. Epub 2016 Jul 14. PMID: 27416522.

ORANGES

Oranges (genus Citrus), with their vibrant colour and tangy flavour, are an excellent source of vitamin C, a vital nutrient needed to support our immune system. Indeed, vitamin C from oranges can also boost the absorption of iron from foods, which aids in protect against anaemia, a common side effect of chemotherapy. Consuming oranges regularly can help in preventing infections and even help decrease the severity and duration of common colds, providing a natural boost to our body's defences. Besides, oranges offer anti-inflammatory benefits, thanks to the presence of bioactive compounds that can help combat inflammation in the body, which can particularly beneficial for individuals experiencing inflammatory conditions or seeking to promote overall wellness. Moreover, blood oranges, a unique variety of oranges, contain higher levels of antioxidants, especially red anthocyanin pigments. These potent antioxidants have been linked to cancer prevention, offering an added layer of health benefits to those who enjoy the distinct flavour and hues of blood oranges. Incorporating oranges into our daily diet can be a delicious and healthful choice, obtaining a generous dose of vitamin C and an array of other bioactive compounds that support our well-being. Whether enjoyed as a refreshing snack, freshly squeezed into juice, or incorporated into various culinary creations, oranges are a delightful way to enhance our health and savour the goodness of nature's bountiful nutrients.

References:

Padayatty SJ, Katz A, Wang Y, et al. Vitamin C as an antioxidant: evaluation of its role in disease prevention. J Am Coll Nutr. 2003 Feb;22(1):18-35. doi: 10.1080/07315724.2003.10719272. PMID: 12569111.

Szeto YT, To TL, Pak SC, et al. A study of DNA protective effect of orange juice supplementation. Appl Physiol Nutr Metab. 2013 May;38(5):533-6. doi: 10.1139/apnm-2012-0344. Epub 2012 Nov 21. PMID: 23668761.

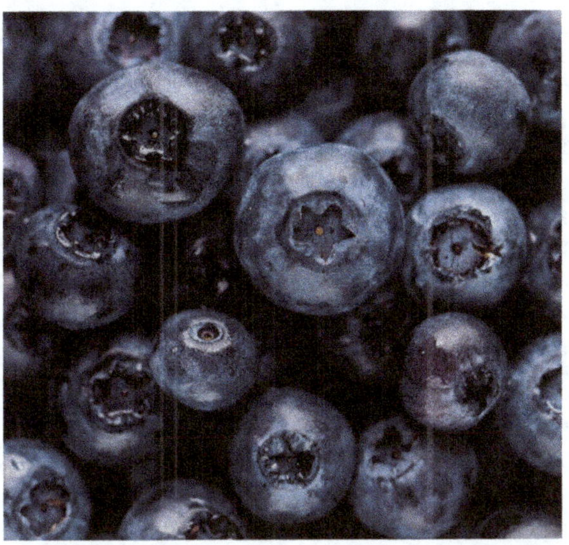

BLUEBERRIES

Blueberries (genus Vaccinium), with their vibrant blue hue and sweet-tart taste, are a true nutritional powerhouse. Bursting with antioxidant compounds, they offer an array of health benefits that make them a delightful addition to our diet. One significant advantage of consuming blueberries is their potential to lower cholesterol levels. Per many studies, the presence of specific compounds in these berries positively impacts cholesterol levels, supporting cardiovascular health and decreasing the risk of heart-related issues. In addition, blueberries help in diabetes prevention, making them a valuable fruit for those seeking to manage blood sugar levels. These little berries also aid in preventing urinary tract infections, as they possess natural compounds that can help protect against bacterial growth in the urinary tract, promoting overall urinary health. Furthermore, blueberries contribute to maintaining healthy eyesight, thanks to the presence of certain bioactive compounds. Furthermore, regular consumption of blueberries has been associated with improved eye health and may help protect against age-related eye diseases.

Notably, other red and dark berries also share similar benefits owing to their richness in anthocyanins and other polyphenols, which have been reported to reduce DNA damage, offering potential protective effects against cellular damage and supporting overall well-being. Hence, incorporating blueberries and a variety of berries into our daily diet is a delightful way to harness the power of nature's antioxidants and nourish our bodies with an abundance of health-promoting nutrients. Whether enjoyed fresh, added to smoothies, or sprinkled over yogurt, these colourful and delicious berries make a flavourful contribution to our quest for optimal health and vitality.

Reference:

Weisel T, Baum M, Eisenbrand G, et al. An anthocyanin/polyphenolic-rich fruit juice reduces oxidative DNA damage and increases glutathione level in health probands. Biotechnol J. 2006 Apr;1(4):388-97. DOI: 10.1002/biot.200600004. PMID: 16892265.

PLUMS

Plums (genus Prunus), with their succulent sweetness and vibrant colours, offer a wealth of health benefits that extend beyond their delightful taste. Abundant in antioxidants, these fruits are champions in safeguarding both the brain and the heart. One of the notable advantages of consuming plums lies in their antioxidant content, which plays a key role in protecting against cancer and promoting eye health. These antioxidants work diligently to combat free radicals and reduce oxidative stress, contributing to overall cellular health and potentially

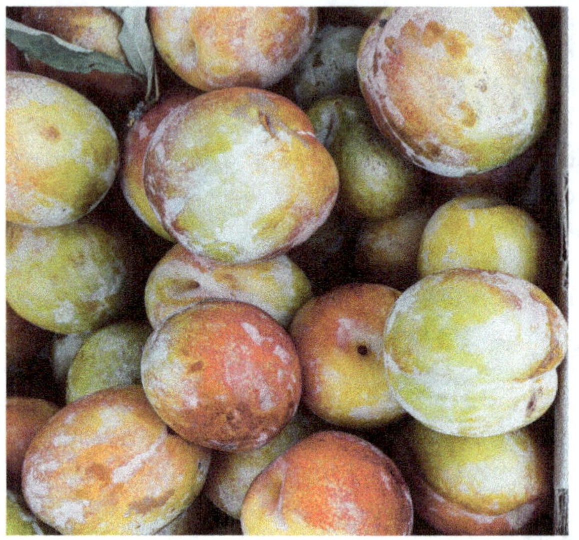

lowering the risk of certain types of cancer. In addition, the presence of specific compounds in plums has been shown to support eye health, making them a valuable addition to promoting excellent vision. Moreover, plums are a good source of iron, a vital mineral that supports healthy blood and overall body maintenance. Adequate iron intake is essential for maintaining optimal energy levels and ensuring the proper functioning of various bodily processes, not to mention combating anaemia caused by chemotherapy.

Remarkably, plums have three times the number of cancer-fighting polyphenols compared with peaches, making them an excellent choice for individuals seeking to enhance their antioxidant intake and strengthen their body's defence against harmful elements. Furthermore, plums contain a carotenoid called lutein, which helps in protecting the brain from damage caused by beta-amyloid fibrils; these fibrils are linked to abnormal angiogenesis found in Alzheimer's disease. The presence of lutein in plums provides a potential means of supporting brain health and mitigating the risk of cognitive decline.

References:

Freedman ND, Park Y, Subar AF, et al. Fruit and vegetable intake and esophageal cancer in a large prospective cohort study. Int J Cancer. 2007 Dec 15;121(12):2753-60. doi: 10.1002/ijc.22993. PMID: 17691111.

Wright ME, Park Y, Subar AF, et al. Intakes of fruit, vegetables, and specific botanical groups in relation to lung cancer risk in the NIH-AARP Diet and Health Study. Am J Epidemiol. 2008 Nov 1;168(9):1024-34. doi: 10.1093/aje/kwn212. Epub 2008 Sep 12. PMID: 18791192; PMCID: PMC2631557.

Katayama S, Ogawa H, Nakamura S. Apricot carotenoids possess potent anti-amyloidogenic activity in vitro. J Agric Food Chem. 2011 Dec 14;59(23):12691-6. doi: 10.1021/jf203654c. Epub 2011 Nov 17. PMID: 22043804.

Erdoğan S, Erdemoğlu S. Evaluation of polyphenol contents in differently processed apricots using accelerated solvent extraction followed by high-performance liquid chromatography-diode array detector. Int J Food Sci Nutr. 2011 Nov;62(7):729-39. doi: 10.3109/09637486.2011.573469. Epub 2011 May 20. PMID: 21599463.

KIWI FRUIT

Kiwi fruit (genus Actinidia) is a powerhouse of health benefits, making it a valuable addition to your diet. Notably, it has the remarkable ability to reduce DNA damage and repair existing damage, thanks to its rich antioxidant content that neutralizes harmful free radicals. In addition, kiwi fruit is a nutrient treasure trove. It provides essential

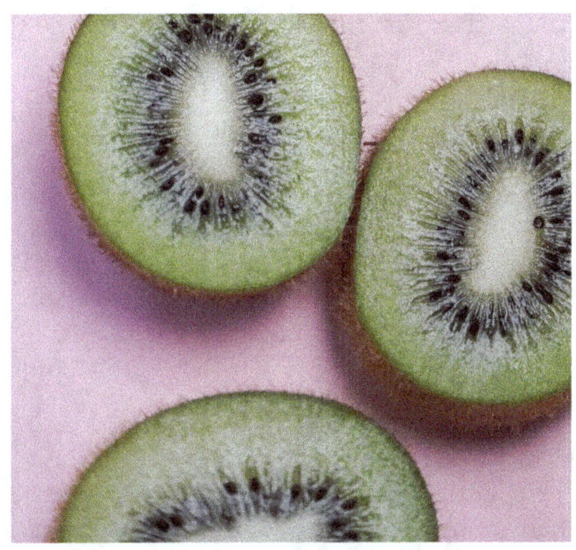

nutrients, such as potassium, copper, vitamin K, folate, and vitamin E, while also being an excellent source of fibre. Its fibre content aids in digestion and can be particularly helpful in relieving constipation.

Moreover, kiwi fruit contains serotonin, a neurotransmitter that contributes to mood regulation and sleep quality. This natural serotonin boost can positively affect both mood and sleep patterns. The benefits don't just stop there. Research has demonstrated that kiwi fruit harbours beneficial gut bacteria, including Lactobacillus and Bifidobacterial—both play a vital role in producing short-chain fatty acids (SCFAs), which support intestinal health and reduce inflammation. Consuming just two kiwi fruits a day can increase the levels of these helpful bacteria in your gut.

By incorporating kiwi fruit into your daily routine, you not only delight your taste buds with its refreshing flavour but also promote a healthier digestive system. The combination of its nutrient content, immune-boosting properties, and gut health support makes kiwi fruit a true superfood, contributing to your overall well-being and vitality. So, why not savour the deliciousness of kiwi fruit and embrace its multitude of health benefits?

References:

Lee YK, Low KY, Siah K, Drummond LM, Gwee KA. Kiwifruit (Actinidia deliciosa) changes intestinal microbial profile. Microb Ecol Health Dis. 2012 Jun 18;23. doi: 10.3402/mehd.v23i0.18572. PMID: 23990838; PMCID: PMC3747767.

Morrison DJ, Preston T. Formation of short chain fatty acids by the gut microbiota and their impact on human metabolism. Gut Microbes. 2016 May 3;7(3):189-200. doi: 10.1080/19490976.2015.1134082. Epub 2016 Mar 10. PMID: 26963409; PMCID: PMC4939913.

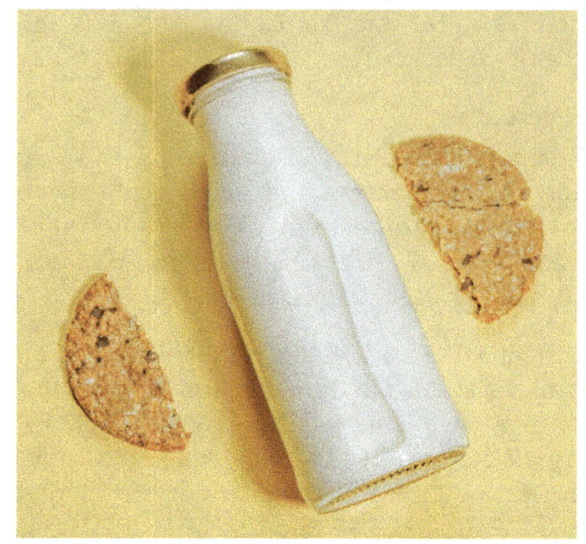

DAIRY

During cancer treatment, it is advisable to opt for non-dairy alternatives to yogurt, milk, and cream, because dairy products can be difficult to digest. However, outside of treatment, consuming full-cream dairy is generally acceptable. Nut-based alternatives, such as brown rice milk, walnut milk, oat milk, coconut milk, almond milk, and cashew milk, are not only easy to digest but also high in calories.

Reference:

Breastcancer.org. Available at www.breast cancer.org/Dietandnutrition/HealthyEating (2022) [Accessed July 27 2023]

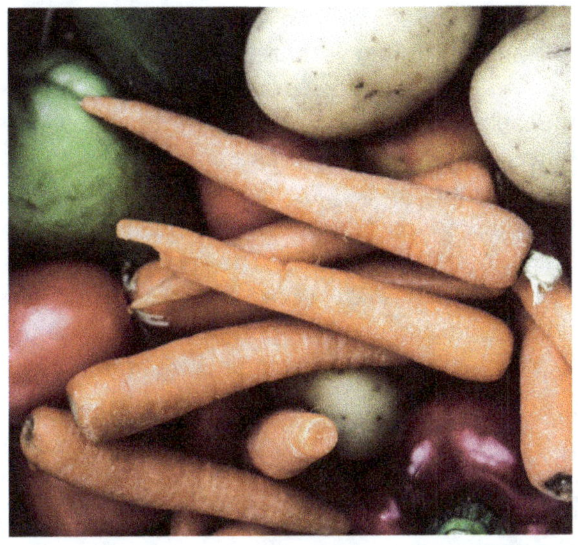

VEGGIES

CARROTS

Carrots (Daucus carota), with their vibrant orange hue and delectable crunch, pack a powerful punch of health benefits, thanks to their abundant carotenes, which play a vital role in promoting overall well-being and supporting various aspects of our health. Rich in beta-carotene, carrots support both day and night vision, helping to enhance visual acuity and support eye health. In fact, beta-carotene converts to vitamin A in the body, a crucial nutrient for maintaining healthy eye function and protecting against age-related vision problems. One of the remarkable advantages of consuming carrots lies in their ability to protect against blood cholesterol and heart disease. Carotenes are known for their heart-healthy properties, as they help reduce cholesterol oxidation, which can lead to the formation of plaques in arteries. By combating this process, carrots contribute to maintaining a healthy cardiovascular system and lowering the risk of heart-related issues.

Furthermore, carrots offer a plethora of essential nutrients, including vitamins, minerals, and fibre, which work in harmony to support various bodily functions, boost immunity, and aid in digestion. Fibre in carrots also contributes to a feeling of fullness, making them a satisfying and healthful addition to our diet. Reportedly, carrots possess the remarkable ability to repair existing DNA damage, which is attributed to the presence of unique compounds in carrots that work to counteract the harmful effects of oxidative stress on our DNA. By assisting in DNA repair, carrots play a role in maintaining cellular health and minimizing the risk of cellular mutations incurred during cancer.

Reference:

Astley SB, Elliott RM, Archer DB, Southon S. Evidence that dietary supplementation with carotenoids and carotenoid-rich foods modulates the DNA damage: repair balance in human lymphocytes. Br J Nutr. 2004 Jan;91(1):63-72. doi: 10.1079/bjn20031001. PMID: 14748939

BRUSSEL SPROUTS

Brussels sprouts (Brassica oleracea, variety gemmifera), the tiny members of the cabbage family, offer diverse health benefits, especially owing to their rich indole content that play a vital role in shielding our body against cancer and impeding its progression, making Brussels sprouts a valuable addition to our diet. Besides their cancer-fighting potential, Brussels sprouts offer a wealth of other advantages for our well-being. They are an excellent source of immune-boosting vitamin

C, which bolsters our body's defences and supports overall immune health. Furthermore, Brussels sprouts are packed with high fibre content, promoting digestive health and regularity. Fibre aids in proper digestion, helps prevent constipation, and supports a healthy gut environment. Hence, incorporating Brussels sprouts into our meals can contribute to a happy and efficient digestive system.

References:

Li Y, Zhang T, Korkaya H, et al. Sulforaphane, a dietary component of broccoli/broccoli sprouts, inhibits breast cancer stem cells. Clin Cancer Res. 2010 May 1;16(9):2580-90. doi: 10.1158/1078-0432.CCR-09-2937. Epub 2010 Apr 13. PMID: 20388854; PMCID: PMC 2862133.

Cohen JH, Kristal AR, Stanford JL. Fruit and vegetable intakes and prostate cancer risk. J Natl Cancer Inst. 2000 Jan 5;92(1):61-8. doi: 10.1093/jnci/92.1.61. PMID: 10620635.

Michaud DS, Spiegelman D, Clinton SK, et al. Fruit and vegetable intake and incidence of bladder cancer in a male prospective cohort. J Natl Cancer Inst. 1999 Apr 7;91(7):605-13. doi: 10.1093/jnci/91.7.605. PMID: 10203279.

Liu X, Lv K. Cruciferous vegetables intake is inversely associated with risk of breast cancer: a meta-analysis. Breast. 2013 Jun;22(3):309-13. doi: 10.1016/j.breast.2012.07.013. Epub 2012 Aug 9. PMID: 22877795.

TOMATOES

Tomatoes (Solanum lycopersicum) are nature's vitamin C powerhouse. As a single medium, tomatoes provide almost a quarter of the recommended daily intake. Beyond this essential nutrient, tomatoes offer an additional advantage—their high potassium content, which aids in maintaining proper body fluid balance. Interestingly, the true potential of tomatoes' nutritional benefits is unleashed through the cooking process. Deep within the tomato cells lies a potent substance called lycopene (a carotenoid). Human body struggles to absorb lycopene efficiently from raw tomatoes. However, the magic happens when tomatoes are cooked, as this process releases and makes lycopene more accessible for our bodies to absorb and utilize effectively.

To maximize lycopene intake, some useful tips come in handy:

Cooking tomatoes in olive oil boosts lycopene absorption by a remarkable three times.

Cherry tomatoes boast a remarkable 24% higher lycopene content compared with other tomato varieties, making them an excellent choice for an extra nutrient boost.

Lycopene's benefits extend far beyond its antioxidant properties. It acts as a shield against free radicals, tackles singlet oxygen, and safeguards our DNA from oxidative damage. These protective actions not only prevent healthy cells from transforming into cancer cells but also support various crucial functions like immune response, cell death regulation, and the activation of enzymes that combat carcinogens. Therefore, embracing the goodness of tomatoes in our diets can be a flavourful way to nourish our bodies and promote overall health and well-being.

References:

Shi J, Le Maguer M. Lycopene in tomatoes: chemical and physical properties affected by food processing. Crit Rev Food Sci Nutr. 2000 Jan;40(1):1-42. doi: 10.1080/1040869 00911 89275. PMID: 10674200.

Unlu NZ, Bohn T, Francis DM, et al. Lycopene from heat-induced cis-isomer-rich tomato sauce is more bioavailable than from all-trans-rich tomato sauce in human subjects. Br J Nutr. 2007 Jul;98(1):140-6. doi: 10.1017/S0007114507685201. Epub 2007 Mar 29. PMID: 17391568.

Bhandari SR, Cho M, Lee JG. Genotypic variation in carotenoid, ascorbic acid, total phenolic, and flavonoid contents, and antioxidant activity in selected tomato breeding lines. Hort Environ Biotechnol. 2016;57:440-52. doi: 10.1007/s13580-016-0144-3

Cooperstone JL, Ralston RA, Riedl KM, et al. Enhanced bioavailability of lycopene when consumed as cis-isomers from tangerine compared to red tomato juice, a randomized, cross-over clinical trial. Mol Nutr Food Res. 2015 Apr;59(4):658-69. doi: 10.1002/mnfr.201400658. Epub 2015 Mar 10. PMID: 25620547; PMCID: PMC4460827.

KIDNEY BEANS

Kidney beans (Phaseolus vulgaris) are an amazing food, abundant in protein, zinc, and fibre, providing essential nutrients for our well-being. Besides, these beans play a vital role in regulating the release of insulin, making them beneficial for maintaining stable blood sugar levels. Besides, these are rich source of antioxidants, making them a must in anticancer diet. Notably, kidney beans should always be cooked before consumption and never eaten raw. Cooking ensures that any potential toxins or harmful substances are neutralized, making the beans safe and enjoyable to eat. Therefore, when preparing kidney beans, take the time to cook them thoroughly to fully savour their nutritional goodness and protect your health. A notable tip here is that you should always soak kidney beans overnight before cooking so as to reduce the cooking time, enhance the texture of cooked beans, reduce bloating & gas after consumption, and ease digestion.

Reference:

Thompson SV, Winham DM, Hutchins AM. Bean and rice meals reduce postprandial glycemic response in adults with type 2 diabetes: a cross-over study. Nutr J. 2012 Apr 11;11:23. doi: 10.1186/1475-2891-11-23. PMID: 22494488; PMCID: PMC3489574.

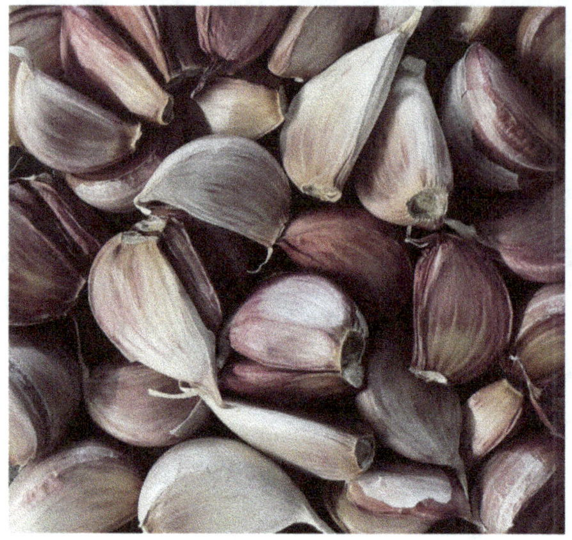

HERBS

GARLIC (Aged Garlic)

Garlic bulbs are truly nature's wonder, boasting powerful antibiotic properties that contribute to reducing the risk of heart disease and cancer. These bulbs hold even more advantages, such as their potent antibiotic effects against fungal infections and their potential to alleviate stomach ulcers. Besides their impressive medicinal qualities, garlic bulbs are a nutritional powerhouse, containing valuable doses of vitamin C, vitamin E, vitamin K, potassium, zinc, iron, magnesium, manganese, and calcium—all essential for overall health. Furthermore, garlic can prevent blood clots and the formation of arterial plaque, promoting a healthy circulatory system. Of note, garlic and onion are natural detoxifiers, which can be beneficial, although they may affect bowel movements. If your child experiences loose bowel movements, it's advisable to avoid these foods until their stools return to normal.

In contrast, aloe vera oil serves as a natural way to harden stools, while peppermint oil can help alleviate constipation. These natural remedies can offer gentle support and balance for your child's digestive system.

Reference:

Nantz MP, Rowe CA, Muller CE, et al. Supplementation with aged garlic extract improves both NK and yǒ-T cell function and reduces the severity of cold and flu symptoms: a randomized, double-blind, placebo-controlled nutrition intervention. Clin Nutr. 2012 Jun;31(3):337-44. doi: 10.1016/j.clnu.2011.11.019. Epub 2012 Jan 24. PMID: 22280901.

BASIL

Basil (Ocimum basilicum), a herb with a rich history of traditional use in easing nausea and stomach aches, has natural anti-inflammatory, antimicrobial, antibacterial, and antimutagenic properties. According to the American Institute for Cancer Research (AICR), basil has abundant flavonoids, which could provide a protective effect against cancer. In fact, its inherent ability to affect viral infections is suggested to contribute to its anticancer properties as well. These beneficial attributes make basil a valuable addition to recipes that not only enhance flavour but also promote overall well-being.

Reference:

Kaefer CM, Milner JA. Herbs and Spices in Cancer Prevention and Treatment. In: Benzie IFF, Wachtel-Galor S, editors. Herbal Medicine: Biomolecular and Clinical Aspects. 2nd edition. Boca Raton (FL): CRC Press/Taylor & Francis; 2011. Chapter 17. Available at https://www.ncbi.nlm.nih.gov/books/NBK92774/

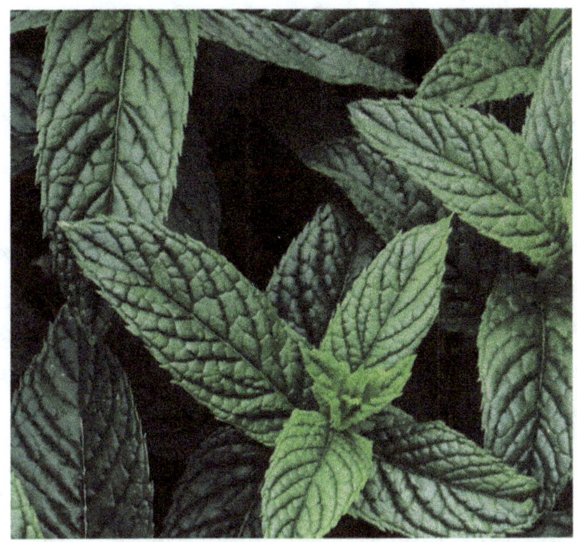

MINT

Mint (genus Mentha), renowned for its soothing effects on the stomach, naturally calms and relaxes digestive discomfort. On top of its digestive benefits, mint boasts antibacterial properties, making it a great addition to promote overall health. Besides, mint's refreshing aroma can help alleviate nasal and chest congestion, making it a versatile and beneficial herb for various purposes. Mint tea or mint candy has been reported to help cancer patients reduce their nausea. Furthermore, a chemical compound in mint, l-menthol, has therapeutic properties that can be beneficial during cancer treatment.

References:

Jafarimanesh H, Akbari M, Hoseinian R, et al. The effect of peppermint (Mentha piperita) extract on the severity of nausea, vomiting and anorexia in patients with breast cancer undergoing chemotherapy: a randomized controlled trial. Integr Cancer Ther. 2020 Jan-Dec;19:1534735420967084. doi: 10.1177/1534735420967084. PMID: 33118401; PMCID: PMC7605047.

Pearson K. 8 health benefits of mint. Healthline. 11 July 2023. Available at https://www.healthline.com/nutrition/mint-benefits

PARSLEY

Parsley (Petroselinum crispum), rich in essential nutrients like vitamin C, potassium, and folate, offers numerous health benefits, such as decreasing fluid retention, assisting in sustaining a healthy fluid balance in the body. Moreover, parsley contains compounds that have the potential to prevent macular degeneration, promoting eye health and well-being. Boasting the highest concentrations of myricetin per 100 g, parsley is suggested to inhibit the cancer-causing effects of heterocyclic amines. In particular, it is an excellent dietary source of apigenine, another flavonoid, as well as folic acid, which could help in preventing cancer. Therefore, adding parsley to your meals can not only enhance flavour but also support your overall health with its nutrient-packed profile.

References:

Tang EL, Rajarajeswaran J, Fung S, et al. Petroselinum crispum has antioxidant properties, protects against DNA damage and inhibits proliferation and migration of cancer cells. J Sci Food Agric. 2015 Oct;95(13):2763-71. doi: 10.1002/jsfa.7078. Epub 2015 Feb 19. PMID: 25582089; PMCID: PMC5024025.

Morales-Brown P. Why is parsley so healthy? 2023. Available at https://www.medicalnewstoday.com/articles/284490 [updated 15 June 2023]

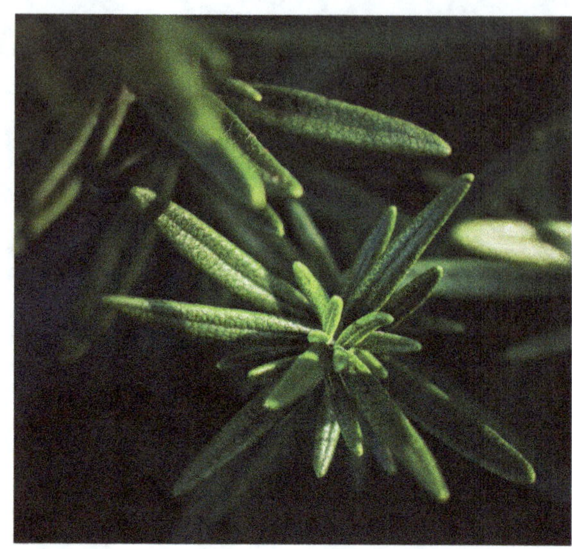

ROSEMARY

Rosemary (Rosmarinus officinalis) is a remarkable herb renowned for its potent antioxidant activity and positive impact on memory and brain function. With its antibacterial and anticancer properties, rosemary also supports overall health and well-being. Recent studies have investigated rosemary for its potential use as a mood lifter, assisting in managing depression. Per the American Institute for Cancer Research (AICR), rosemary is rich in a phytochemical called carnosol, which has been shown to slow cancer cell growth, boost immune functions, and hinder the production of cancer-related hormones. Hence, embracing the aromatic and flavourful essence of rosemary in your dishes can not only augment your culinary experience but also contribute to a healthier and happier you.

Reference:

Kaefer CM, Milner JA. Herbs and Spices in Cancer Prevention and Treatment. In: Benzie IFF, Wachtel-Galor S, editors. Herbal Medicine: Biomolecular and Clinical Aspects. 2nd edition. Boca Raton (FL): CRC Press/Taylor & Francis; 2011. Chapter 17. Available at www.ncbi.nlm.nih.gov/books/NBK92774/

THYME

Thyme (genus Thymus), a prized herb, holds a prominent position among culinary choices owing to its essential oils that possess robust antibacterial properties, safeguarding against food poisoning bugs. Notably, thyme offers more benefits beyond its culinary uses. Thyme helps boost omega-3 levels, promoting heart health and overall well-being. Its consumption has been correlated with enhanced brain power and cognitive function. Rich in antioxidants, vitamin C, and iron, and several active agents, such as apigenin, thymol, tannins, carvacrol, luteolin, and other oils, thyme contributes to a nutritious diet and supports immune health. Thus, embracing thyme in your meals not only adds delightful flavours but also introduces a range of health-enhancing properties to your plate.

Reference:

Kaefer CM, Milner JA. Herbs and Spices in Cancer Prevention and Treatment. In: Benzie IFF, Wachtel-Galor S, editors. Herbal Medicine: Biomolecular and Clinical Aspects. 2nd edition. Boca Raton (FL): CRC Press/Taylor & Francis; 2011. Chapter 17. Available at www.ncbi.nlm.nih.gov/books/NBK 92774/

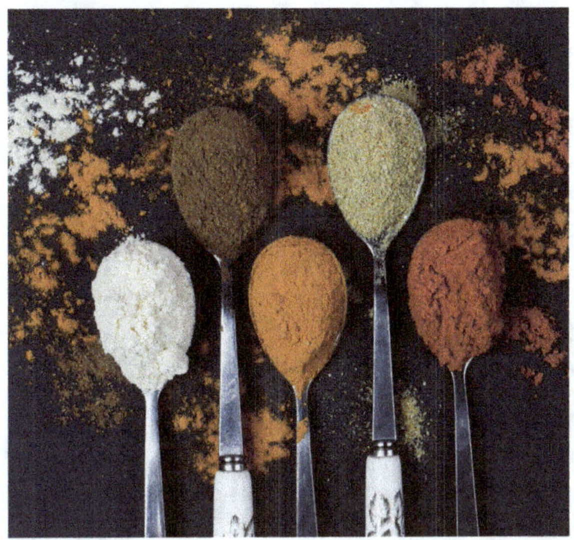

SPICES

CINNAMON

Cinnamon (genus Cinnamomum), a fragrant and flavourful spice, offers more than just its delightful taste. With its anti-inflammatory and antibacterial properties, cinnamon serves as a valuable addition to our diet, helping in digestion and reducing bloating. Other advantages of cinnamon include its antibacterial and antifungal properties, which contribute to overall well-being, potential prevention of blood clots, and promoting heart health and circulation. Among various beneficial phytonutrients present in cinnamon, eugenol has been reported to directly kill certain types of cancer cells. Hence, embracing cinnamon in cancer patients' diet not only adds a pleasant aroma and taste but also help in alleviating the side effects of chemotherapy.

Reference:

Kaefer CM, Milner JA. Herbs and Spices in Cancer Prevention and Treatment. In: Benzie IFF, Wachtel-Galor S, editors. Herbal Medicine: Biomolecular and Clinical Aspects. 2nd edition. Boca Raton (FL): CRC Press/Taylor & Francis; 2011. Chapter 17. Available at www.ncbi.nlm.nih.gov/books/NBK92774/

CUMIN

Cumin (Cuminum cyminum) seeds, known for their distinct flavour, offer numerous health benefits. They are not only aid in digestion but also possess antiseptic properties. The iron content in cumin seeds contributes to maintaining healthy blood levels. Creating an infusion of cumin seeds with honey in a warm drink can effectively soothe sore throats, making it a natural and comforting remedy. Specifically, thymo-quinone in black cumin seed oil has antimicrobial, anti-inflammatory, antioxidant, and chemopreventive properties. In some scientific experiments, cumin has demonstrated the potential to inhibit cancer cell proliferation. Thus, embracing the use of cumin seeds in your culinary repertoire can be a flavourful way to support your overall well-being.

Reference:

Kaefer CM, Milner JA. Herbs and Spices in Cancer Prevention and Treatment. In: Benzie IFF, Wachtel-Galor S, editors. Herbal Medicine: Biomolecular and Clinical Aspects. 2nd edition. Boca Raton (FL): CRC Press/Taylor & Francis; 2011. Chapter 17. Available at www.ncbi.nlm.nih.gov/books/NBK92774/

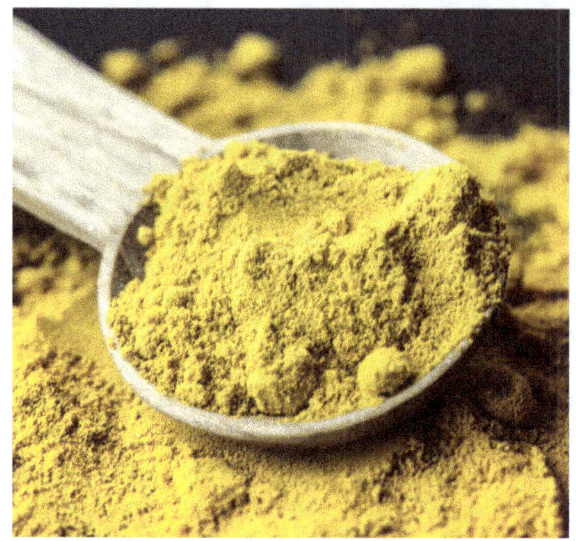

TURMERIC

Turmeric (genus Curcuma), a magical spice with healing properties, offers a wide array of health benefits that make it a true superfood for our well-being. Not only is it a powerful anti-inflammatory spice but also it holds the potential for combating cancer and improving our blood cholesterol profile. At the heart of turmeric's wonders lies its main bioactive component, curcumin, which not only exhibits anti-inflammatory effects but also exerts epigenetic effects that safeguard the health of our blood vessels. Research has indicated that consuming turmeric could kill cancer cells and even stop tumours from forming the blood vessels they need to grow. However, there is also a notable downside of this spice. Turmeric has been reported to exert some potential side effects in cancer patients, such as increased bleeding from affecting platelets. Hence, its consumption during cancer treatment comes with the certified nutritionist's discretion.

Considering the many challenges our children's delicate blood vessels face, such as frequent poking and exposure to chemicals, the protective role of turmeric becomes even more significant. For instance, my own son had encountered difficulties with collapsed and weak veins, causing difficulties in drawing blood. This damage, accumulated over time, has prompted us to use an ultrasound machine for locating a suitable vein, even five years after the initial challenges.

Useful Tip: # When using turmeric, add a little black pepper. It will help your body absorb the benefits of turmeric better.

Reference:

What Are the Benefits of Turmeric — and Can It Be Used to Prevent or Treat Cancer? Here's What the Science Says. Available at https://www.mskcc.org/news/what-are-benefits-turmeric-and-can-it-be-used-prevent-treat-cancer-here-s-what-science-says [cited October 27, 2021].

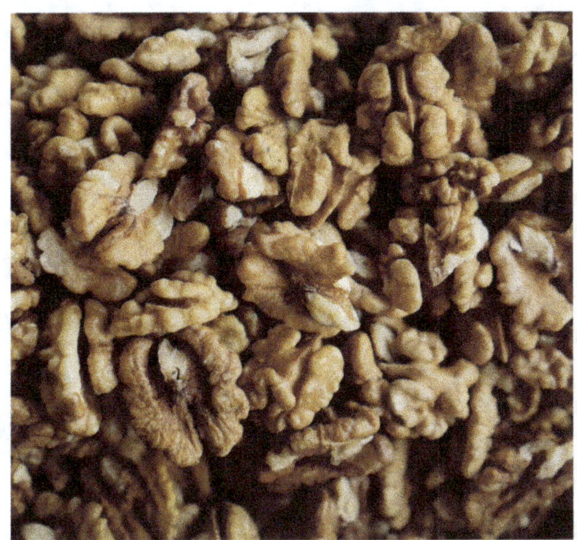

References:

Bamberger C, Rossmeier A, Lechner K, et al. A walnut-enriched diet affects gut microbiome in healthy Caucasian subjects: a randomized, controlled trial. Nutrients. 2018 Feb 22;10(2):244. doi: 10.3390/nu10020244. PMID: 29470389; PMCID: PMC5852820.

Hardman WE. Walnuts have potential for cancer prevention and treatment in mice. J Nutr. 2014 Apr;144(4 Suppl):555S-560S. doi: 10.3945/jn.113.188466. Epub 2014 Feb 5. PMID: 24500939; PMCID: PMC3952627.

DRY FRUITS

WALNUTS

Walnuts (genus Juglans) are a nutritional powerhouse, packed with essential nutrients like omega-3 fatty acids, polyunsaturated fats (PUFA), and dietary fibre. Incorporating walnuts into your diet can significantly reduce the risk of various health conditions, ranging from cardiovascular diseases to certain types of cancer. Research has shown that consuming just 21 walnut halves daily can positively influence gut health because walnuts can increase the abundance of beneficial bacteria, such as Bifidobacterial and Firmicutes, in the gut, which play a crucial role in producing anti-inflammatory short-chain fatty acids (SCFA) such as butyrate, propionate, and acetate. By enjoying a handful of walnuts each day, you not only nourish your body with essential nutrients but also promote a healthier gut environment, which contributes to overall well-being.

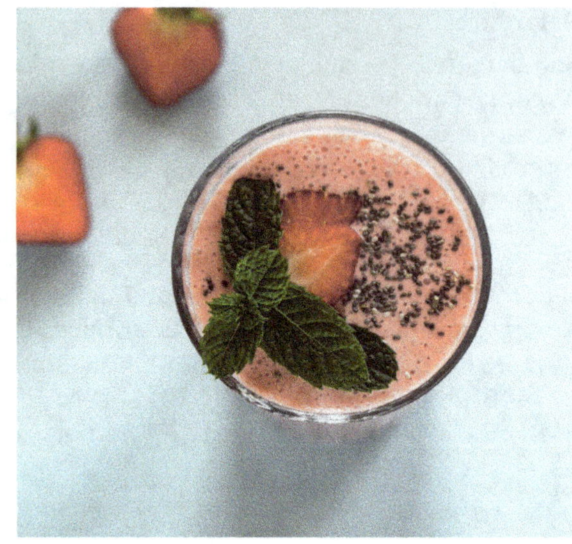

DRINKS

COCONUT WATER

Coconut water, a refreshing and hydrating drink, is an excellent source to maintain our body's electrolyte balance. Embracing coconut water offers a host of benefits, including:

- reducing the production of harmful free radicals, supporting our overall health;

- providing faster rehydration compared with regular water, making it an ideal choice for replenishing fluids after physical activities; and

- potentially alleviating feelings of nausea and soothing stomach discomfort, making it a soothing option for digestion.

Thus, enjoying the natural goodness of coconut water not only quenches our thirst but also provides essential advantages that keep us feeling revitalized and well-nourished. Coconut water may not be everyone's favourite taste, especially for children. However, for children who rely on an NG tube for nutrition and hydration, coconut water can be a wonderful option to ensure they stay well-hydrated. By administering coconut water through the tube, parents can provide their children with the benefits of this hydrating beverage even if they have difficulty consuming it orally. Besides, its ability to maintain electrolyte balance and offer faster rehydration makes it a valuable addition to their nutritional support, helping them stay nourished and hydrated with the goodness of coconut water.

References:

Geetha V, Kumar GS. Concentrates from tender coconut water and coconut testa beneficially modulates tissue lipid profiles in high-fat fed rats. J Food Sci Technol. 2022 Apr;59(4):1649-1657. doi: 10.1007/s13197-021-05178-2. Epub 2021 Jul 21. PMID: 35250088; PMCID: PMC8882753.

Alleyne T, Roache S, Thomas C, et al. The control of hypertension by use of coconut water and mauby: two tropical food drinks. West Indian Med J. 2005 Jan;54(1):3-8. doi: 10.1590/s0043-31442005000100002. PMID: 15892382.

Mohamad NE, Yeap SK, Abu N, et al. In vitro and in vivo antitumour effects of coconut water vinegar on 4T1 breast cancer cells. Food Nutr Res. 2019 Jan 10;63. doi: 10.29219/fnr.v63.1616. PMID: 30814922; PMCID: PMC6387426.

JUICE

Incorporating nourishing sun-protective juice can be a valuable addition to the diet of children undergoing cancer treatment. Did you know that tomato, watermelon, guava, and pink grapefruit are packed with lycopene, a powerful antioxidant? So, these juices not only taste delicious but can also work wonders for your skin. Studies have revealed that sipping on a shot of these juices about an hour before heading outdoors can provide natural protection from the sun's harmful rays. It's like a shield of defence for your skin, especially if you are on medication that makes your skin more sensitive to sunlight.

References:

Weisel T, Baum M, Eisenbrand G, et al. An anthocyanin/polyphenolic-rich fruit juice reduces oxidative DNA damage and increases glutathione level in healthy probands. Biotechnol J. 2006 Apr;1(4):388-97. doi: 10.1002/biot.200600004. PMID: 16892265.

Takahashi S, Hamasuna R, Yasuda M, et al. A randomized clinical trial to evaluate the preventive effect of cranberry juice (UR65) for patients with recurrent urinary tract infection. J Infect Chemother. 2013 Feb;19(1):112-7. doi: 10.1007/s10156-012-0467-7. Epub 2012 Sep 8. PMID: 22961092.

Nantz MP, Rowe CA, Muller C, et al. Consumption of cranberry polyphenols enhances human gd-T cell proliferation and reduces the number of symptoms associated with colds and influenza: a randomised, placebo-controlled intervention study. Nutr J. 2013 Dec 13;12:161. doi: 10.1186/1475-2891-12-161. PMID: 24330619; PMCID: PMC3878739.

Yoo YM, Jang SK, Kim GH, et al. Pharmacological advantages of melatonin in immunosenescence by improving activity of T lymphocytes. J Biomed Res. 2016 Jul;30(4):314-21. doi: 10.7555/JBR.30.2016K0010. Epub 2016 May 20. PMID: 27533940; PMCID: PMC4946322.

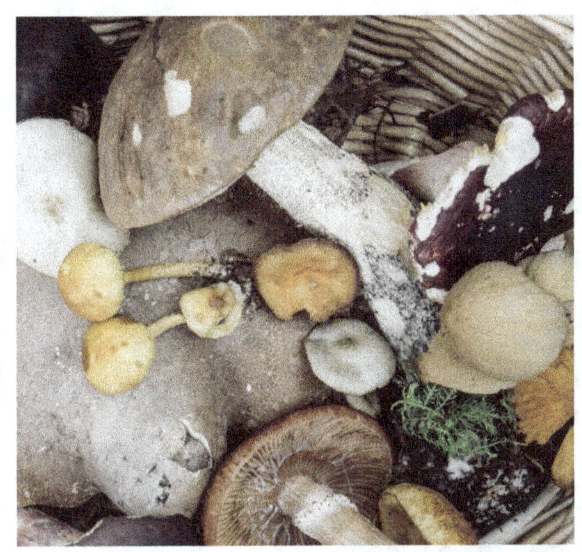

MUSHROOMS

White button mushrooms (Agaricus bisporus) are a valuable source of bioactive compounds, predominantly beta-glucan, which is known for its immune-stimulating properties. The consumption of mushrooms activates the gut, igniting a chain reaction that stimulates the immune system to produce antibodies, which then play a crucial role in defending the body against harmful pathogens and invaders, bolstering the body's natural defence mechanisms. With their immune-boosting benefits, mushrooms serve as a delicious and nutritious addition to your diet, contributing to overall health and well-being. Hence, incorporating white button mushrooms into your meals can support your immune system and help keep you feeling strong and protected.

References:

Rossouw W, Korsten L. Cultivable microbiome of fresh white button mushrooms. Lett Appl Microbiol. 2017 Feb;64(2):164-170. doi:

10.1111/lam.12698. PMID: 27930823.

Varshney J, Ooi JH, Jayarao BM, et al. White button mushrooms increase microbial diversity and accelerate the resolution of Citrobacter rodentium infection in mice. J Nutr. 2013 Apr;143(4):526-32. doi: 10.3945/jn.112.171355. Epub 2013 Jan 23. PMID: 23343678; PMCID: PMC3738246.

Jeong SC, Koyyalamudi SR, Pang G. Dietary intake of Agaricus bisporus white button mushroom accelerates salivary immunoglobulin A secretion in healthy volunteers. Nutrition. 2012 May;28(5):527-31. doi: 10.1016/j.nut.2011.08.005. Epub 2011 Nov 23. PMID: 22113068.

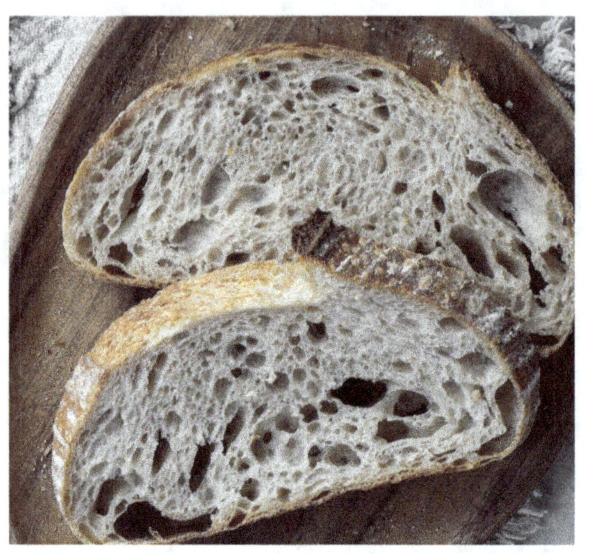

SOURDOUGH BREAD

In the process of making sourdough bread, live bacteria known as Lactobacillus reuteri (a type of probiotic bacteria) are used. This bacterium is remarkable for its various health functions. Studies have demonstrated that L. reuteri can boost immunity, inhibit tumour growth, and even accelerate wound healing. In addition, antioxidants, such as peptides, in sourdough have been reported to decrease the risk for cardiovascular diseases, Alzheimer's, other chronic illnesses related to inflammation, and certain types of cancer. Compared with other bread types, sourdough bread exerts a relatively less effect on blood sugar and insulin levels, thereby having a lower glycaemic index. Unlike many bacteria that perish during the heating or cooking of food, L. reuteri leaves behind beneficial bacterial fragments that remain in the baked sourdough bread, which have been found to retain their health benefits, making sourdough bread not only delicious but also a potentially advantageous addition to our diet.

References:

Mu Q, Tavella VJ, Luo XM. Role of Lactobacillus reuteri in human health and disease. Front Microbiol. 2018 Apr 19;9. https://doi.org/10.3389/fmicb.2018.00757

Lakritz JR, Poutahidis T, Levkovich T, et al. Beneficial bacteria stimulate host immune cells to counteract dietary and genetic predisposition to mammary cancer in mice. Int J Cancer. 2014 Aug 1;135(3):529-40. doi: 10.1002/ijc.28702. Epub 2014 Jan 10. PMID: 24382758; PMCID: PMC4131439.

Varian BJ, Poutahidis T, DiBenedictis BT, et al. Microbial lysate upregulates host oxytocin. Brain Behav Immun. 2017 Mar;61:36-49. doi: 10.1016/j.bbi.2016.11.002. Epub 2016 Nov 5. PMID: 27825953; PMCID: PMC5431580.

DARK CHOCOLATE

Dark chocolate offers a delightful combination of health benefits that go beyond satisfying your sweet tooth. Rich in cacao, it contains compounds that have anti-angiogenic and stem cell–stimulating properties, which can contribute to overall well-being. In addition, the cacao present in dark chocolate has been reported to exert positive effects on gut microbiota, promoting a healthy balance of beneficial bacteria in the digestive system. However, that's not all—indulging in dark chocolate can also favourably affect your mental health. Some studies have suggested that consuming dark chocolate may help reduce feelings of anxiety by lowering stress markers in the body. For cancer patients, the American Cancer Society recommends eating a high-quality dark chocolate with at least 70% cocoa. Hence, treating yourself to a

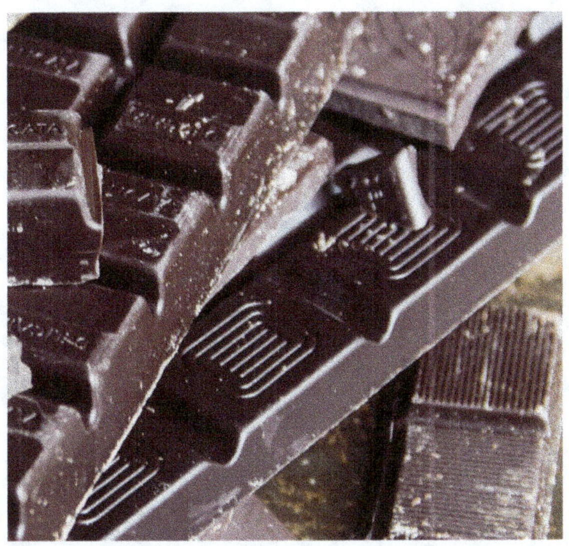

square of dark chocolate not only pleases your taste buds but also supports your gut and mind, making it a truly enjoyable and beneficial treat.

Martin FP, Rezzi S, Peré-Trepat E, et al. Metabolic effects of dark chocolate consumption on energy, gut microbiota, and stress-related metabolism in free-living subjects. J Proteome Res. 2009 Dec;8(12):5568-79. doi: 10.1021/pr900607v. PMID: 19810704.

NOURISHING SUPPORT

STRATEGIES FOR FEEDING, SNACKING AND HYDRATION DURING TREATMENT

FOOD PRESENTATION: UNLEASH YOUR CULINARY CREATIVITY

Get ready to elevate your food presentation skills and unleash your inner MasterChef. Transforming your meals into visually appealing and enticing creations doesn't have to be time-consuming or complicated. It's all about stimulating the senses, especially when one of our children's senses may be a little off. Let's focus on engaging their sense of smell and sight.

Here are some amazing tips to take your plating to the next level:

EMBRACE SMALLER PLATES: Opt for smaller plates to create an illusion of abundance and make the dish look more visually satisfying.

PLAY WITH DIFFERENT SHAPES: Experiment with various plate shapes to add visual interest and create unique presentations that stand out.

AMP UP THE APPEAL: Make your meals look irresistible and intriguing. Spice up ordinary dishes by using cookie cutters to create fun and appealing shapes.

EMBRACE LAYERS AND HEIGHTS: Play with different layers and heights to add depth and dimension to your presentation. Stacking elements or arranging them at varying heights can make the dish visually captivating.

VIBRANT COLOURS: Incorporate bright and vibrant colours into your dishes. For example, you can make rainbow pasta using natural colour dyes, which adds a playful and eye-catching element to the plate. Given below are some of the safest food colouring sources:

- Beetroot and tomatoes (Red)
- Strawberries and Raspberries (Pink)
- Saffron and turmeric (Yellow)
- Carrots, sweet potatoes, and paprika (Orange)
- Matcha and spinach (Green)
- Blueberries and purple sweet potato (Purple)

Remember, food presentation is an art that allows you to express your creativity and enhance the overall dining experience. Therefore, have fun, let your imagination soar, and create visually stunning masterpieces that will delight both the eyes and taste buds of your loved ones.

SAFER KITCHEN, SAFER MEALS:
ITEMS TO REMOVE FROM YOUR KITCHEN

Create a safer and healthier cooking environment by identifying and removing potential hazards from your kitchen. Discover the importance of eliminating certain plastics, non-stick cookware, and other potentially unsafe materials.

NON-STICK PANS: A WORD OF CAUTION

It's best to avoid non-stick pans made with Teflon (a synthetic chemical prepared from carbon and fluorine atoms) as they can easily overheat. When the coating reaches high temperatures, it releases toxic fumes known as polymer fume fever, which can be harmful to the lungs. Hence, choose safer alternatives (e.g., utensils made of cast iron, stainless steel, ceramic, glass, and enamel-coated cast iron) to ensure a healthier cooking experience.

PLASTIC STORAGE CONTAINERS

Be mindful of plastic storage containers, as they can break down over time, contaminating food with potentially harmful chemicals. Instead, opt for glassware to store leftovers to avoid any risk of contamination. Moreover, refrain from reheating food in plastic containers, as this process can increase the leaching of chemicals into your food. Bear in mind that the label "microwave safe" only indicates that the container won't melt in the microwave; it doesn't guarantee that it's free from chemical leaching. Therefore, prioritise using safer materials, such as glass, to ensure the safety and quality of your stored and reheated food.

PLASTIC AND STYROFOAM UTENSILS AND TOOLS

Replace your plastic spatulas, spoons, colanders, and measuring cups with safer alternatives (such as those made of stainless steel, food-grade silicone, and wood), as they can release chemicals into your food when exposed to heat. In particular, avoid cookware made of plastic, nylon, melamine, and non-stick Teflon. Switching to non-plastic options will ensure that your cooking utensils do not release harmful substances into your meals, promoting a healthier and safer cooking environment.

PLASTIC DRINK BOTTLES AND BOTTLED WATER

It is highly recommended to avoid storing or drinking water from plastic bottles because of the potential ingestion of harmful chemicals. Plastic containers can release chemicals like BPA (Biphenyl A), which acts as an estrogen mimic in the body and could contribute to health issues like diabetes, obesity, fertility problems, behavioural disorders, and early puberty in girls. Moreover, leaving plastic drink bottles in cars or under the sun can result in the release of another chemical called "dioxin" into the water. Several studies have linked dioxin exposure to an elevated risk of breast cancer. To safeguard our health, go for safer alternatives, such as glass, copper, and steel bottles, and avoid using plastic bottles for water storage or consumption.

REFERENCE:

VoPham T, Bertrand KA, Jones RR, et al. Dioxin exposure and breast cancer risk in a prospective cohort study. Environ Res. 2020 Jul;186:109516. doi: 10.1016/j.envres.2020.109516. Epub 2020 Apr 13. PMID: 32305677; PMCID: PMC7363533.

NOURISHING BOLUS FOOD IDEAS FOR ENTERAL FEEDING

Enteral feeding, also known as bolus feeding and tube feeding, is a method of feeding where a specific amount of liquid nutrition is delivered directly into the stomach or small intestines through a feeding tube at set intervals throughout the day. When tube feeding is provided in the hospital setting, it is termed as enteral nutrition (EN), whereas when it occurs outside the hospital setting, it is termed as home enteral nutrition (HEN). When planning bolus feeds, it's essential to consider the nutritional needs of the individual and any dietary restrictions they may have. Given below are some food ideas suitable for bolus feeding:

BLENDERISED MEALS: Blend together cooked and soft foods until smooth consistency is attained that can easily pass through the feeding tube. Some options include:

- pureed vegetables (e.g., carrots, peas, and sweet potatoes);
- pureed fruits (e.g., bananas, apples, and pears); and
- cooked meats (e.g., chicken, turkey, and beef) blended with broth or gravy for added moisture and flavour.

SOUPS AND STEWS: Prepare well-cooked and blended soups and stews with a balanced mix of proteins, vegetables, and grains.

SMOOTHIES: Create nutritious smoothies by blending fruits, vegetables, yogurt, milk, protein powder, and other supplements as needed.

NUTRITIONAL SUPPLEMENTS: Commercially available nutrition supplements specifically designed for enteral feeding can be used to meet specific dietary requirements.

RICE OR GRAIN PORRIDGE: Cook rice, oats, or other grains until soft and blend them with water or milk for a smooth consistency.

APPLESAUCE OR MASHED BANANAS: These soft and easily digestible fruits can be blended to a smooth texture.

YOGURT: Opt for plain, smooth yogurt (e.g., Greek yogurt) without chunks or fruit pieces. Yogurt is an excellent dietary source of conjugated linoleic acid (CLA), iodine, and calcium, as well as some riboflavin and vitamin B12.

HUMMUS: A pureed mixture of chickpeas, tahini, lemon juice, and garlic can provide a good source of protein and healthy fats. As it is prepared from anti-inflammatory ingredients, such as chickpeas, olive oil, and sesame seeds, hummus is highly beneficial for cancer patients. Adding a little turmeric, enriches its anti-inflammatory and healing properties.

LENTIL OR BEAN PUREE: Cooked lentils (e.g., red lentils) or beans can be blended into a smooth puree and seasoned with herbs and spices.

SCRAMBLED EGGS: Soft scrambled eggs can be blended for a protein-rich option.

PUMPKIN PUREE

PREP TIME: 15 minutes (preparing the pumpkin and assembling) | COOKING TIME: 45-60 minutes (baking the pumpkin) | TOTAL TIME: 1-1.25 hours (including baking and cooling time)

SERVING: Approximately 2-3 cups of pumpkin puree, depending on the pumpkin size. The number of servings may vary based on portion sizes, but it's roughly enough for about 8-12 small servings of baby food.

INGREDIENTS	METHOD
1 small pumpkin (approximately 1 kg) Water	Preheat your oven to 200°C (390°F) [fan-forced]. Wash the pumpkin thoroughly and cut it in half. Scoop out the seeds and discard them. Place the pumpkin halves on a baking tray, cut side up. Fill the tray with about 1-2 cm (approximately 1/2 inch) of water. Cover the tray with aluminium foil and bake the pumpkin in the preheated oven for about 45-60 minutes, or until the pumpkin is soft and tender. Once the pumpkin is cooked, let it cool slightly. Scoop out the flesh from the pumpkin skin and transfer it to a blender or food processor. Blend the pumpkin until a smooth puree is obtained. You can add a little water or breast milk/formula to attain the desired consistency. Serve the pumpkin puree warm or refrigerate it for 3 days in an airtight container for later use. It can be served as a standalone puree or mixed with other pureed fruits or vegetables.

VEGETABLE BROTH

PREP TIME: 10-15 minutes (chopping and assembling ingredients) | COOKING TIME: 45 minutes to 1 hour (simmering the broth) | TOTAL TIME: Approximately 55 minutes to 1.25 hours (including simmering and cooling time)

SERVING: Approximately 6 cups of vegetable broth. The number of servings may vary based on portion sizes, but it's roughly enough for about 6-8 servings of broth.

INGREDIENTS:

2 carrots, washed and roughly chopped

2 celery stalks, washed and roughly chopped

1 onion, peeled and roughly chopped

2 garlic cloves, peeled

1 bay leaf

6 cups water

INSTRUCTIONS:

In a large pot, combine the chopped carrots, celery, onion, garlic, and bay leaf.

Pour in the water and bring the mixture to a boil over medium-high heat.

Once it starts boiling, reduce the heat to low, cover the pot with a lid, and let it simmer for about 45 minutes to 1 hour. This will allow the flavours to infuse into the broth.

After simmering, remove the pot from the heat and let it cool slightly.

Strain the broth through a fine mesh strainer into a clean bowl or container, discarding the solids.

Let the vegetable broth cool completely before transferring it to airtight containers for storage (3 days).

-Any vegetables can be used, the more colourful the better.

HEALTH BENEFITS

NUTRIENT RETENTION: Steaming vegetables preserves more nutrients than other cooking methods like boiling or frying. Drinking the leftover water provides a nutrient-rich broth containing vitamins, minerals, and antioxidants released from the vegetables during the steaming process.

HYDRATION: Vegetable broth is a liquid, contributing to your overall hydration. Staying properly hydrated is crucial for supporting various bodily functions and promoting overall well-being.

DIGESTIVE HEALTH: The vegetable broth contains soluble fibre that aids in digestion and promotes a healthy gut. It can also help prevent constipation and support a well-functioning digestive system.

LOW-CALORIE OPTION: Typically, vegetable broth is low in calories, making it a suitable choice for those looking to maintain a healthy weight or reduce caloric intake.

ENHANCED FLAVOUR: The leftover water from steamed vegetables is rich in flavour, especially if the vegetables were seasoned during the steaming process. It adds depth and taste to soups, stews, sauces, and various dishes.

IMMUNE SUPPORT: The vitamins and antioxidants present in vegetable broth can support your immune system and help protect against illnesses.

To make the most of the benefits, use a variety of colourful vegetables to ensure a diverse range of nutrients in your vegetable broth. You can enjoy the broth as a nourishing drink, use it as a base for soups or sauces, or incorporate it into your cooking to enhance the flavour of your dishes. However, be cautious with the amount of salt or seasoning used during steaming, as excessive sodium intake should be avoided. Embrace this simple and healthy practice to elevate your culinary experience and promote wellness.

FUELLING THE FIGHT: HIGH-CALORIE SNACKS FOR YOUNG CANCER WARRIORS

When considering high-calorie snacks for children with cancer, it's important to prioritise nutrient-dense options that provide essential vitamins and minerals while being easily digestible. Given below are some high-calorie snack ideas that can benefit paediatric patients with cancer:

NUT BUTTER AND FRUIT: Spread almond butter, peanut butter, or cashew butter on apple slices, banana, or whole-grain crackers.

AVOCADO TOAST: Mash avocado on whole-grain toast and sprinkle with a pinch of salt and pepper for added flavour.

CHEESE AND CRACKERS: Serve whole-grain crackers with slices of cheese for a protein and calorie boost.

TRAIL MIX: Create a calorie-dense trail mix with nuts, seeds, dried fruits, and a few chocolate chips for a sweet touch.

GREEK YOGURT PARFAIT: Layer Greek yogurt with granola and mixed berries to make a delicious and nutrient-packed snack.

SMOOTHIES: Blend together fruits, milk/yogurt, nut butter, and a dash of honey for a high-calorie, nutrient-rich beverage.

CHEESE QUESADILLAS: Make mini quesadillas with whole-grain tortillas and cheese for a tasty and calorie-dense snack.

MINI SANDWICHES: Prepare small sandwiches with whole-grain bread, lean protein (e.g., turkey and chicken), and avocado or cheese.

RICE CAKES WITH TOPPINGS: Top rice cakes with cream cheese, avocado, or hummus for added calories.

ENERGY BITES: Mix oats, nut butter, honey, and add-ins like dried fruits and chocolate chips to create calorie-packed energy bites.

PUDDING CUPS: Choose high-protein and high-calorie pudding cups made with whole milk or fortified with protein.

MUFFINS: Bake homemade muffins with added nuts, seeds, and dried fruits for extra calories.

BANANA SPLITS: Create a healthier version of a banana split by topping a banana with yogurt, nuts, and a drizzle of honey.

MINI CHEESE PIZZA: Make small, whole-grain English muffin or pita bread pizzas topped with cheese and veggies.

MINI PANCAKES OR WAFFLES: Prepare small pancakes or waffles using whole-grain flour and serve with a dollop of nut butter or Greek yogurt.

NOURISHING TINY TUMMIES: ESSENTIAL NUTRIENTS FOR BABIES IN TREATMENT

BABIES (AGE: 4-6 MONTHS)

For babies aged 4-6 months, introducing solid foods should be done with caution and under the guidance of a paediatrician, especially if the baby is undergoing cancer treatment. At this age, babies are typically just beginning their journey into solid foods through the process of weaning. Here are some gentle and appropriate baby food ideas for this age range group:

SINGLE GRAIN CEREALS: Start with iron-fortified single grain cereals, such as rice cereal or oatmeal, mixed with breast milk or formula to attain a smooth and runny consistency.

PUREED FRUITS: Offer smooth and well-cooked pureed fruits, such as apples, pears, bananas, and avocados. These should be introduced one at a time to check for any potential allergies.

PUREED VEGETABLES: Introduce single-ingredient pureed vegetables, such as sweet potatoes, carrots, peas, and squash. Again, introduce them one by one to monitor for allergies.

BABY RICE OR OATMEAL PORRIDGE: Prepare homemade rice or oatmeal porridge using breast milk or formula to create a gentle and nutritious meal.

APPLESAUCE: Provide unsweetened applesauce as a natural and soothing option.

MASHED BANANAS: Offer mashed bananas, which are easy to digest and a good source of nutrients.

PUMPKIN PUREE: Introduce smooth pumpkin puree for added variety.

BABY YOGURT: Choose plain, whole-milk yogurt without added sugars or artificial flavours.

STEAMED AND PUREED CHICKEN OR TURKEY: If the paediatrician recommends introducing meat, provide well-cooked and pureed chicken or turkey.

VEGETABLE BROTH: Offer homemade vegetable broth to provide hydration and a mild taste.

Remember to introduce new foods one at a time and wait for a few days before introducing another new food, as this helps to identify any potential allergies or sensitivities. During cancer treatment, the baby's immune system could be compromised, so it's crucial to prioritise hygiene and food safety while preparing and offering baby food.

BABIES (AGE: 6-12 MONTHS)

For babies aged 6-12 months undergoing cancer treatment, their nutritional needs may evolve as they continue to grow and develop. During this stage, you can introduce a wider variety of foods to support their health and provide essential nutrients. Here are some baby food ideas suitable for babies in this age group:

SOFT COOKED VEGETABLES: Offer soft-cooked vegetables, such as carrots, peas, sweet potatoes, broccoli, and zucchini. Ensure that they are cooked until tender and easy to mash.

FRUITS: Introduce a variety of mashed or pureed fruits, including bananas, apples, pears, peaches, and blueberries.

BABY CEREALS: Continue with iron-fortified baby cereals, such as rice, oatmeal, or mixed grain cereals, which provide essential nutrients.

PROTEIN-RICH FOODS: Offer pureed or mashed sources of protein, such as well-cooked chicken, turkey, beef, or lentils.

DAIRY PRODUCTS: Introduce plain, full-fat yogurt or cottage cheese, which provides calcium and protein.

AVOCADO: Mash avocado for healthy fats and essential nutrients.

EGG YOLK: Gradually introduce well-cooked and mashed egg yolk, which is a good source of iron.

PASTA AND RICE: Offer well-cooked and soft pasta and rice dishes for added variety.

SMOOTHIES: Create nutrient-rich smoothies by blending fruits, yogurt, and a little spinach or kale for added nutrients.

NUT BUTTERS: Offer smooth nut butters, such as almond or peanut (if there are no nut allergies), as a source of healthy fats and protein.

MASHED POTATOES: Serve mashed potatoes with added breast milk or formula for extra creaminess.

PUMPKIN OR BUTTERNUT SQUASH SOUP: Continue with mild and creamy pumpkin or butternut squash soup.

SOFT CHEESE: Introduce soft and easily spreadable cheeses like cream cheese or ricotta.

FISH: If recommended by the paediatrician, offer well-cooked and mashed fish like salmon or cod.

VEGETABLE AND CHICKEN BROTH: Prepare a light vegetable and chicken broth to provide hydration and nourishment.

Remember to introduce new foods one at a time and watch for any allergic reactions or sensitivities. In addition, ensure the baby is appropriately supervised during meals and feeding. Always consult with the baby's paediatrician and oncology team before introducing any new foods or making changes to their diet, especially during cancer treatment. They will be able to provide personalized advice and recommendations based on the baby's health condition and specific needs.

MANAGING ASPIRATION

Aspiration is defined as accidental inhalation of any foreign object or substance into your airway. In a medical setting, aspiration can occur when using a nasogastric (NG) tube—a medical device inserted through the nose and down the throat into the stomach to deliver nutrition, fluids, or medications to individuals who cannot consume these substances orally.

Aspiration with an NG tube can be caused because of the following:

IMPROPER PLACEMENT: If the NG tube is not correctly positioned into the stomach, it may enter the respiratory tract, leading to the accidental inhalation of fluids or contents intended for the stomach into the lungs.

TUBE DISLODGMENT: The NG tube may become displaced or move from its intended position, increasing the likelihood of aspiration.

REFLEX ACTIONS: Coughing, gagging, or other reflexes can cause the contents of the NG tube to be expelled into the airway instead of reaching the stomach.

VOMITING: In cases of vomiting while the NG tube is in place, there is a risk of aspirating the vomit into the lungs.

Aspiration through an NG tube can have serious consequences, such as aspiration pneumonia and respiratory distress. To minimize the risk, healthcare professionals take precautions by ensuring proper NG tube placement and monitoring patients for signs of aspiration or tube displacement. When long-term enteral feeding is necessary or there is a higher risk of aspiration, healthcare providers may consider alternative feeding methods, such as surgically placed gastrostomy (G-tube) or jejunostomy (J-tube) tubes directly into the stomach or small intestines. If someone using an NG tube experiences symptoms of aspiration, such as coughing, difficulty breathing, or fever, immediate medical attention should be sought for proper evaluation and management.

PREVENTION METHODS WE USED

MAINTAINING UPRIGHT POSITION: Whenever possible, we ensured that Jake stayed in an upright position while being fed through the NG tube. This practice helped minimize the risk of aspiration and provided a more comfortable feeding experience.

POST-FEEDING UPRIGHT TIME: After each feed, we kept Jake in an upright position for around 30-60 minutes. Not only did this help in preventing aspiration but also we noticed a positive impact on reducing reflux episodes.

Elevating the Bed: For overnight feedings at home, we elevated the top of Jake's bed. We achieved this by using additional pillows or blankets placed under the mattress. To ensure a more stable incline, we found that a wedge foam pillow from Clark Rubber worked best. Unlike regular pillows that tend to flatten over time, the wedge foam maintained its shape throughout the 3 years we used it.

HOW TO CHECK NG TUBE PLACEMENT BEFORE FEEDING

CONFIRM PRESCRIPTION AND CHILD'S IDENTITY: Check the NG tube insertion prescription provided by the healthcare team and ensure you have the correct child by verifying their name and date of birth.

HAND HYGIENE: Wash your hands thoroughly with soap and water or use a hand sanitizer before handling the NG tube.

GATHER EQUIPMENT: Ensure you have the necessary equipment ready, including a stethoscope, a syringe (usually 5–10 mL), and pH indicator strips (optional).

POSITION THE CHILD: Position the child in an upright or semi-upright position, which helps facilitate the proper passage of the NG tube into the stomach.

MEASURE TUBE LENGTH: Measure the length of the exposed NG tube outside the child's nose. Check if it aligns with the initial insertion measurement.

CHECK FOR RESPIRATORY PLACEMENT: Use the stethoscope to listen for breath sounds over the child's stomach and lung areas. The absence of lung sounds over the stomach indicates correct placement in the stomach.

CHECK FOR GASTRIC ASPIRATION: Connect the syringe to the end of the NG tube and gently aspirate gastric contents. Observe the volume and colour of the aspirate. Gastric aspirate usually appears acidic, with a pH level of 1-5.

OPTIONAL STEP FOR PH VERIFICATION: 8. Check pH Level (optional): If pH indicator strips are available, apply a small amount of gastric aspirate to the strip and match the colour change to the pH chart. A pH level of 1-5 confirms gastric placement.

SECURE THE TUBE: After confirming proper placement, secure the NG tube to the child's nose using tape or a tube holder to prevent unintended dislodgment.

DOCUMENT THE VERIFICATION: Record the NG tube verification procedure, noting the time, confirmation method, aspirate characteristics, and any child response.

For further information and specific considerations, you can refer to the Royal Children's Hospital Melbourne guidelines: "Nasogastric Tube Insertion and Verification." The Royal Children's Hospital Melbourne (https://www.rch.org.au/clinicalguide/guideline_index/ Nasogastric_Tube_Insertion_and_Verification/).

Remember to always consult with the healthcare team if you have any doubts about the NG tube's placement or if the child shows signs of discomfort, distress, or respiratory issues during the feeding process.

Flushing an NG tube is a critical procedure to maintain its patency and prevent blockages. The process involves using a syringe to gently push a prescribed liquid through the tube. Follow these steps based on the general guidelines:

ITEMS NEEDED

A 10-20 mL syringe (size may vary depending on the NG tube).

Sterile water or normal saline, as prescribed by the healthcare professional.

STEPS

HAND HYGIENE: Thoroughly wash your hands with soap and water or use a hand sanitizer before handling the NG tube and syringe.

POSITION THE CHILD: Place the child in an upright or semi-upright position to minimize the risk of aspiration and facilitate flushing.

CHECK PLACEMENT: Before flushing, ensure the NG tube is correctly positioned in the child's stomach. Follow the recommended verification steps to confirm placement.

PREPARE THE SYRINGE: Draw the prescribed amount of sterile water or normal saline into the syringe, per healthcare professional's instructions.

CONNECT THE SYRINGE: Attach the syringe to the NG tube's end connected to the child's nose.

FLUSH THE TUBE: Slowly and gently push the syringe plunger to instil the sterile water or saline into the NG tube. Ensure the liquid flows smoothly.

OBSERVE FOR RESISTANCE OR BLOCKAGE: If you encounter resistance or difficulty during flushing, stop immediately, and do not force the flush. Contact the healthcare team for further guidance.

REMOVE THE SYRINGE: Once the flush is complete, carefully disconnect the syringe from the NG tube.

DOCUMENT THE PROCEDURE: Record the flushing procedure, noting the time, amount of liquid used, and any observations made during the process.

Of note, flushing frequency and the volume of liquid used may vary based on individual patient needs and healthcare professional recommendations. Always adhere to the healthcare team's instructions regarding NG tube flushing to ensure the child's safety and well-being.

TIPS BASED ON OUR EXPERIENCE

During Jake's time with an NG tube, we discovered a helpful trick to prolong the tube's life and ease the traumatic experience for him. As his tube started to develop a milky white residue from his night feeds, we found a simple method to clean it effectively. First, we added 10 mL of cola (coke) into the tube and let it sit for a few minutes. The cola's properties broke down the film that had built up within the tube. Then, gently rolling and squeezing the tube further aided in removing the residue. Next, to ensure thorough cleaning, we flushed the tube with 10 mL of water. Furthermore, we kept a small amount of water in the tube to maintain its patency and prevent clogging. By using this technique periodically, we managed to extend the tube life and ensure it remained clear, providing Jake with a more comfortable feeding experience. As always, it's essential to consult with healthcare professionals for guidance and support when caring for an NG tube.

Notably, during Jake's time with the NG tube, we discovered a technique called the "push and pull method" to clear potential blockages. However, this method proved to be challenging for him as it made him gag, leading to the accidental dislodgment of the NG tube on some occasions. Hence, we decided to use this method sparingly. The push and pull method involves introducing fluid into the tube and then withdrawing it to dislodge any obstructions. While it can be effective in some cases, it may not be suitable for all children, especially those who are sensitive or prone to gagging.

TOTAL PARENTERAL NUTRITION (TPN) FOR CHILDREN UNDERGOING CANCER TREATMENT

Total parenteral nutrition (TPN) is a specialized medical treatment in which essential nutrients, including carbohydrates, proteins, fats, vitamins, and minerals, are delivered directly into a child's bloodstream through an intravenous (IV) line. TPN is used when a child is unable to obtain sufficient nutrition through their digestive system, either because of their medical condition or as a result of cancer treatment.

For children undergoing cancer treatment, TPN serves several crucial purposes:

NUTRITIONAL SUPPORT: Cancer and cancer treatments, such as chemotherapy or radiotherapy, often lead to reduced appetite, swallowing difficulties, or gastrointestinal issues, which can hinder a child's ability to consume adequate nutrition through regular meals.

MAINTAINING NUTRITIONAL STATUS: Proper nutrition is essential for a child's growth, development, and immune function. During cancer treatment, sustaining optimal nutritional status is crucial to support overall health and enhance the child's ability to cope with treatment side effects.

ADDRESSING MALNUTRITION: Cancer treatment can result in malnutrition, where the body lacks essential nutrients for proper functioning. TPN delivers the necessary nutrients directly into the bloodstream, preventing malnutrition and related complications.

MINIMIZING TREATMENT DELAYS: By ensuring that children receive adequate nutrition through TPN, it may help prevent treatment delays due to inadequate nutrition or treatment-related side effects.

ENHANCING TREATMENT TOLERANCE: Adequate nutrition can improve a child's tolerance to cancer treatment, allowing them to undergo the full course of therapy with fewer disruptions.

SUPPORTING HEALING AND RECOVERY: TPN provides the energy and nutrients needed for healing, recovery, and tissue repair during and after cancer treatment.

TPN administration is performed under the careful supervision of a specialized healthcare team, including paediatric oncologists, nutritionists, and nurses. The composition of the TPN solution is tailored to fulfill the specific nutritional needs of each child based on their medical condition and treatment requirements. It is essential to closely monitor the use of TPN to prevent complications and ensure the child's overall well-being. The healthcare team will regularly assess the child's progress and make adjustments to the TPN regimen as necessary.

TRANSITIONING FROM TPN TO ORAL FEEDING: A STEP-BY-STEP GUIDE

The process of transitioning a child from TPN to oral feeding is a vital step in their cancer treatment journey. This phase encompasses gradually reintroducing oral feedings while simultaneously decreasing reliance on TPN. The transition warrants careful planning, close monitoring, and a collaborative effort between the healthcare team and the child's family. Here's an overview of the step-by-step guide for a successful transition:

ASSESSMENT AND PREPARATION: The healthcare team methodically assesses the child's readiness for oral feeding. Factors like improved appetite, bowel function, and overall health are carefully evaluated.

START SMALL: The transition begins with the introduction of small amounts of easily digestible and well-tolerated foods, such as clear liquids, broths, or diluted fruit juices. These are added to the child's existing TPN regimen.

GRADUAL INCREASE IN ORAL VOLUME: Over time, the quantity of oral feedings is slowly increased, while the TPN is slowly reduced. The healthcare team closely monitors the child's tolerance to the increasing volume of oral intake.

ENSURING ADEQUATE NUTRITION AND CALORIES: Throughout the transition, the healthcare team ensures that the child receives sufficient nutrition and calories from both oral feedings and TPN to support growth, development, and energy needs.

BALANCING ORAL AND PARENTERAL NUTRITION: A delicate balance is maintained between oral and parenteral nutrition to meet the child's unique nutritional requirements. The healthcare team makes adjustments as needed per the child's progress.

ADDRESSING CHALLENGES: Challenges such as feeding aversions, taste fluctuations, or gastrointestinal issues may arise during the transition. The healthcare team provides support and strategies to address these challenges effectively.

REGULAR MONITORING AND NUTRITION SUPPORT: Continuous monitoring of the child's weight, growth, and nutritional status is essential throughout the transition process. The healthcare team ensures appropriate nutritional support and promptly addresses any concerns.

INVOLVEMENT OF A DIETITIAN: A paediatric dietitian plays a decisive role in creating a personalized diet plan, considering the child's preferences, food allergies, and dietary restrictions.

FAMILY EDUCATION AND SUPPORT: The child's family is educated about the transition process, including the significance of adhering to the diet plan and recognizing signs of successful oral feeding progression.

GRADUAL TPN WEANING: As the child's oral intake improves, the TPN is slowly tapered down. The healthcare team closely monitors the child's response and adjusts the TPN weaning process accordingly.

ATTAINING ORAL FEEDING INDEPENDENCE: The ultimate goal of the transition is for the child to attain full oral feeding independence, with minimal or no reliance on TPN.

ONGOING FOLLOW-UP CARE: After accomplishing oral feeding independence, the child continues to receive regular follow-up care to ensure sustained nutrition and address any nutritional concerns that may arise.

The transition from TPN to oral feeding is individualized for each child, considering their unique medical condition and response to treatment. The healthcare team provides unwavering guidance, support, and encouragement to both the child and their family during this journey, with the ultimate aim of achieving optimal nutrition and overall well-being.

TIPS BASED ON OUR EXPERIENCE

During your child's time on TPN, they may experience frequent and extremely loose bowel movements. The consistency of the stool can be liquid or have a mucus-like appearance, resembling gastroenteritis symptoms. Given the various medications, chemotherapy, blood transfusions, oxygen support, and pain relief they receive, it can be challenging for them to reach the toilet in time. As a helpful tip during hospital stays or extended medical care, consider purchasing a supply of inexpensive underwear and make sure to bring extra pairs. This way, you can easily dispose of any soiled underwear, reducing the burden of laundry and maintaining hygiene during this challenging time. Besides, this precaution serves as a safety measure, as loose bowel movements may contain traces of chemotherapy, requiring proper management to minimize exposure. By adopting this approach, you can enhance your child's comfort and manage the challenges associated with loose bowel movements during TPN treatment. Remember to keep the healthcare team informed about any concerns or changes in your child's condition to receive appropriate guidance and support.

MANAGING EXCESSIVE HUNGER (HYPERPHAGIA)

Hyperphagia (polyphagia) is a feeling of extreme, insatiable hunger, which could occur in patients undergoing cancer treatment. You can manage hyperphagia as follows:

BALANCED MEALS: Focus on providing balanced meals that include a mix of carbohydrates, proteins, and healthy fats to promote satiety.

FIBRE-RICH FOODS: Including foods high in fibre can help keep a child feeling fuller for longer.

REGULAR MEAL SCHEDULE: Establishing a regular meal schedule can help regulate hunger and prevent excessive snacking.

HEALTHY SNACK OPTIONS: Offer nutritious snack options that are satisfying and help control hunger between meals.

In this regard, communication and support also play a key role. It is essential to communicate openly with the child about their appetite and food preferences. Encourage them to express their feelings and concerns related to eating during treatment. Providing emotional support, understanding, and patience can create a positive environment for mealtimes.

MAINTAINING HYDRATION DURING CHILDHOOD CANCER TREATMENT: ENCOURAGING FLUID INTAKE AND ADDRESSING DEHYDRATION

It is crucial for children undergoing cancer treatment to stay hydrated as it supports their overall health, helps manage treatment side effects, and aids in their recovery. Cancer treatments, such as chemotherapy and radiotherapy, can lead to various factors that may exacerbate the risk of dehydration. This chapter emphasizes the significance of hydration and explores effective ways to encourage fluid intake and prevent dehydration risks.

IMPORTANCE OF HYDRATION DURING CANCER TREATMENT

SUPPORTING TREATMENT TOLERANCE: Staying hydrated helps the body tolerate cancer treatments better, reducing the chances of treatment interruptions or delays.

PREVENTING DEHYDRATION: Cancer treatments can cause side effects like nausea, vomiting, diarrhoea, or increased sweating, leading to fluid loss and potential dehydration.

PROMOTING OVERALL WELL-BEING: Proper hydration contributes to better energy levels, reduced fatigue, and overall well-being during the child's cancer journey.

STRATEGIES TO ENCOURAGE FLUID INTAKE

OFFERING A VARIETY OF BEVERAGES: Provide a range of appealing beverages, such as water, diluted fruit juices, herbal teas, and clear broths, to make drinking enjoyable.

USING FUN AND COLOURFUL CUPS: Use colourful and age-appropriate cups or bottles to make drinking more exciting, especially for younger children.

INCLUDING FLUID-RICH FOODS: Incorporate foods with high water content, such as watermelon, cucumbers, oranges, and soups, into the child's diet.

SETTING HYDRATION REMINDERS: Set reminders for regular drinking throughout the day, especially during or after cancer treatments.

ENSURING ACCESSIBILITY: Ensure that the child always has easy access to water or beverages, whether at home, in the hospital, or during outings.

ICY POLES AND ICE CHIPS: Offer popsicles or ice chips to keep the child hydrated, especially if they experience mouth sores or difficulties in drinking fluids.

RECOGNIZING DEHYDRATION SIGNS: Educate caregivers about the signs of dehydration, such as dry mouth, dark urine, lethargy, and dizziness, so they can promptly address any concerns.

MONITORING FLUID INTAKE: Keep track of the child's daily fluid intake to ensure they are meeting their hydration needs.

REPLACING FLUID LOSSES: In case of vomiting or diarrhoea, work with the healthcare team to replace lost fluids adequately.

OFFERING ELECTROLYTE SOLUTIONS: In severe dehydration or electrolyte imbalances, the healthcare team may recommend oral rehydration solutions to restore fluid and electrolyte balance.

SEEKING MEDICAL ATTENTION: If signs of dehydration are observed or the child has difficulty drinking sufficient fluids, seek immediate medical attention for appropriate intervention.

FAMILY AND CAREGIVER SUPPORT

Involving the entire family and caregivers in maintaining the child's hydration creates a positive and supportive environment. Thus, encourage open communication about fluid intake, hydration goals, and any challenges faced.

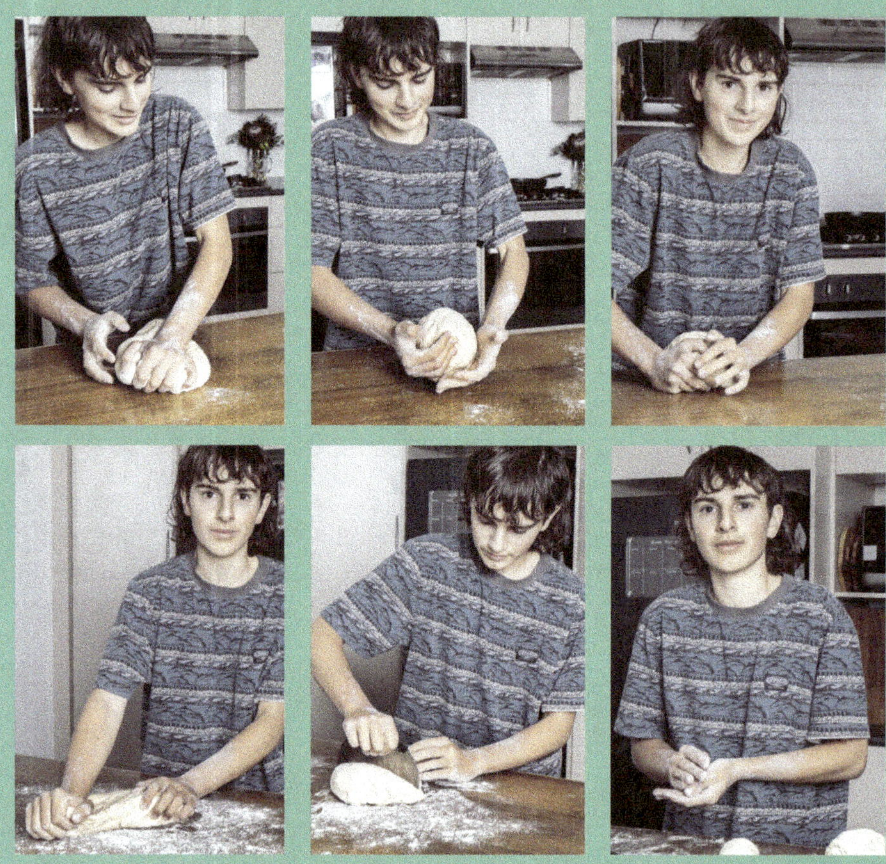

TASTE & THRIVE

This chapter provides some recipes to enhance your child's well-being while undergoing cancer treatment.

TOMATO SAUCE

PREP TIME 15 minutes (chopping and assembling ingredients)

COOKING TIME 25–30 minutes (cooking the sauce)

TOTAL TIME Approximately 40-45 minutes

INGREDIENTS

1 tbsp olive oil

1 small onion, chopped

2-3 garlic cloves, crushed

1 small celery stick, finely chopped

1 bay leaf

450 g ripe tomatoes, peeled and chopped

1 tbsp tomato puree, blended with 150 mL of water

A few sprigs of fresh oregano

Pepper, to taste

METHOD

Heat the oil in a heavy-based saucepan. Add onion, garlic, celery, and bay leaf. Gently sauté, stirring frequently, for 5 minutes.

Stir in tomatoes and blended tomato puree. Season with pepper to taste and add oregano. Bring to a boil, then reduce the heat, cover, and simmer, stirring occasionally, for 20-25 minutes, until the tomatoes have completely collapsed. If you prefer a thicker sauce, simmer for an additional 20 minutes.

Discard the bay leaf and oregano. Transfer the mixture to a food processor and blend until a chunky puree is formed. Taste and adjust the seasoning if necessary.

NOTE: This tomato sauce is perfect for pasta dishes, pizzas, or as a base for other recipes. Store any leftovers in an airtight container in the refrigerator for 3-5 days.

SERVING: Approximately 2 cups of tomato sauce. The number of servings may vary based on portion sizes, but it's roughly enough for about 4 servings, depending on how you're using it.

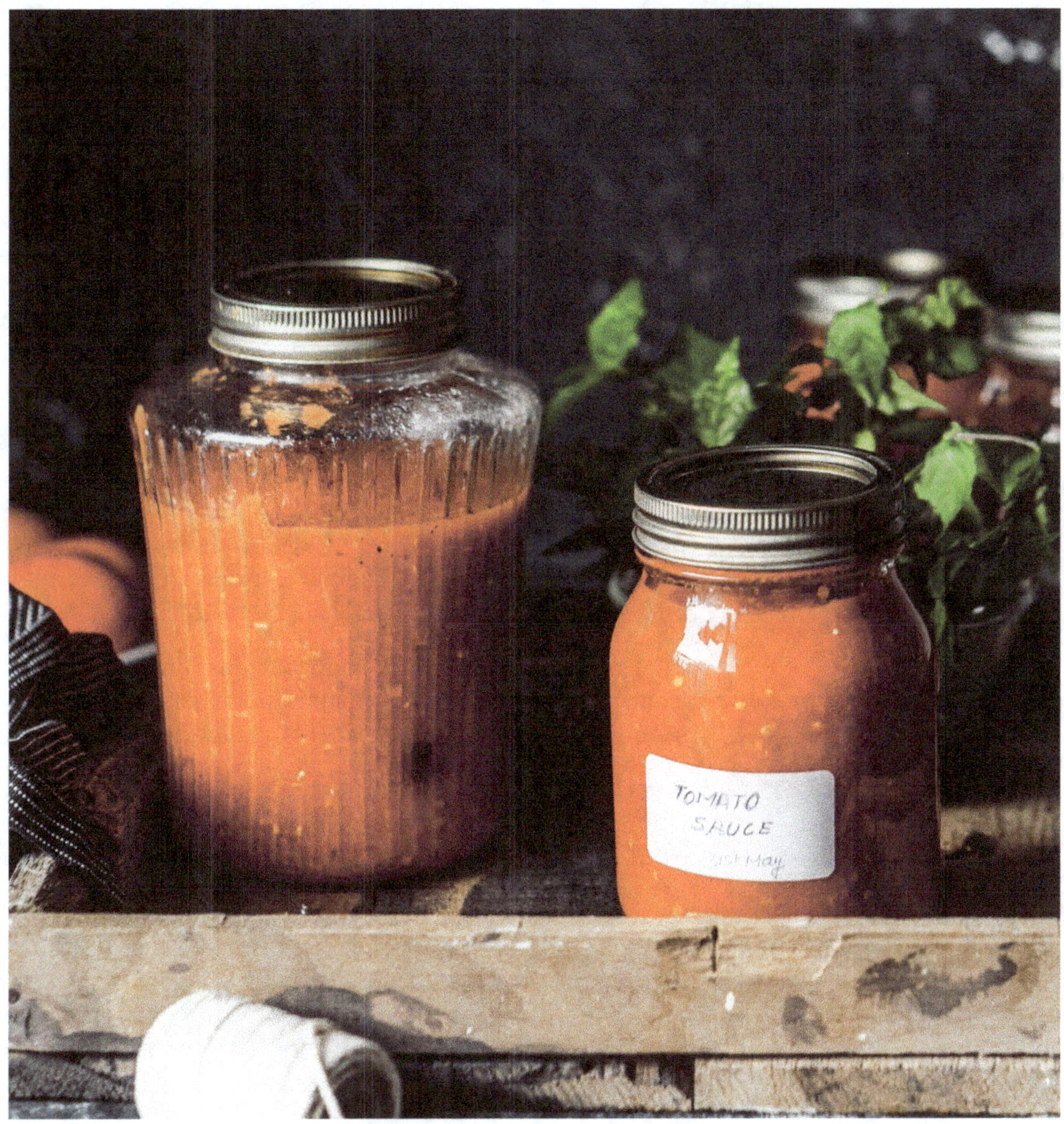

NUTRITIONAL INFORMATION: Calories: 53 kcal | Carbohydrates: 6 g | Protein: 7 g | Fat: 1 g | Saturated Fat: 1 g | Trans Fat: 0 g | Cholesterol: 3 mg | Sodium: 24 mg | Potassium: 126 mg | Fibre: 1 g | Sugar: 4 g | Vitamin A: 10 IU | Vitamin C: 3 mg | Calcium: 77 mg | Iron: 1 mg

THYME, ROSEMARY, AND LEMON OIL

PREP TIME 15-20 minutes (preparing the ingredients)

COOKING TIME 1.5-2 hours (heating the oil in the oven)

TOTAL TIME Approximately 1.75-2.25 hours (including heating and cooling time)

INGREDIENTS

10-15 fresh thyme sprigs

5 fresh rosemary sprigs

Zest of 2 lemons

250 mL rapeseed oil

METHOD

Preheat the oven to 150°C/300°F (fan-forced). Remove leaves from thyme and rosemary sprigs. Cut the lemon zest into strips.

Pour rapeseed oil into an ovenproof glass dish and add thyme leaves, rosemary leaves, and lemon zest strips. Place the dish in the centre of the preheated oven and heat for 1.5-2 hours.

If you have a digital thermometer, test the oil. It should reach a temperature of 120°C/250°F before you remove it from the oven. Leave the oil to cool for at least 30 minutes. Store the oil in the refrigerator as it is or strain it through a muslin cloth.

NOTE: This fragrant thyme, rosemary, and lemon oil is perfect for adding depth of flavour to various dishes. Use it as a marinade, drizzle it over roasted vegetables, or add it to dressings and sauces. The oil can be stored in a sealed jar in the refrigerator for up to 2 weeks.

NUTRITIONAL INFORMATION Calories: About 2000-2200 kcal (mainly from the oil) | Carbohydrates: Negligible (mainly from the lemon zest) | Protein: Negligible | Fibre: Negligible | Sodium: Negligible | Fat: Approximately 224-245 g (depending on the oil used)

TURMERIC PASTE

PREP TIME 5-10 minutes (measuring and mixing the ingredients)

COOKING TIME None

TOTAL TIME 5-10 minutes

INGREDIENTS

1/4 cup turmeric powder

1/4 cup coconut oil

1 tsp freshly ground black pepper

1 tsp ground ginger

1/2 tsp cinnamon

METHOD

In a small saucepan over medium heat, combine turmeric powder, coconut oil, black pepper, ground ginger, and cinnamon.

Stir the mixture consistently until it forms a smooth paste. Remove the saucepan from the heat.

Whisk in the virgin coconut oil, black pepper, ground ginger, and cinnamon until well combined.

Transfer the paste to a glass jar and store it in the refrigerator for up to 2 weeks.

NOTE: Turmeric paste is a convenient way to incorporate the health benefits of turmeric into your daily routine. You can add it to curries, soups, smoothies, or warm milk. The added fat from the coconut oil aids in turmeric absorption, and the black pepper enhances its bioavailability. Enjoy the anti-inflammatory properties and the delicious flavour this paste brings to your dishes.

NUTRITIONAL INFORMATION: Calories: About 340-360 kcal | Carbohydrates: About 18-20 g | Protein: About 1-2 g | Fibre: Around 3-4 g | Sodium: Negligible | Fat: Approximately 28-30 g

GUT HEALTH SOUP
SLOW COOKER RECIPE

PREP TIME 15-20 minutes (chopping and assembling ingredients) |

COOKING TIME 6-8 hours on low or 3-4 hours on high (slow cooking the soup) |

TOTAL TIME Approximately 6.25-8.25 hours (including prep and slow cooking time)

INGREDIENTS

1 litre bone broth

1 butternut pumpkin, chopped into cubes

3 large potatoes, chopped into cubes

1 large sweet potato, chopped into cubes

1 can coconut milk

1 tsp turmeric

1 tsp ginger

1/2 tsp pepper

Pink salt, to taste

Mixed herbs

2 sticks celery, chopped

METHOD

Place all the ingredients, except for coconut milk, into a slow cooker.

Cook on low heat until the vegetables are soft and cooked through.

Once cooked, add coconut milk to the slow cooker.

Use a blender to blend the soup until smooth and creamy.

Serve the soup warm and store any excess in an airtight container in the refrigerator for up to a week. It can also be frozen for later use.

SERVING: Approximately 4-6 servings of gut health soup, depending on the serving size.

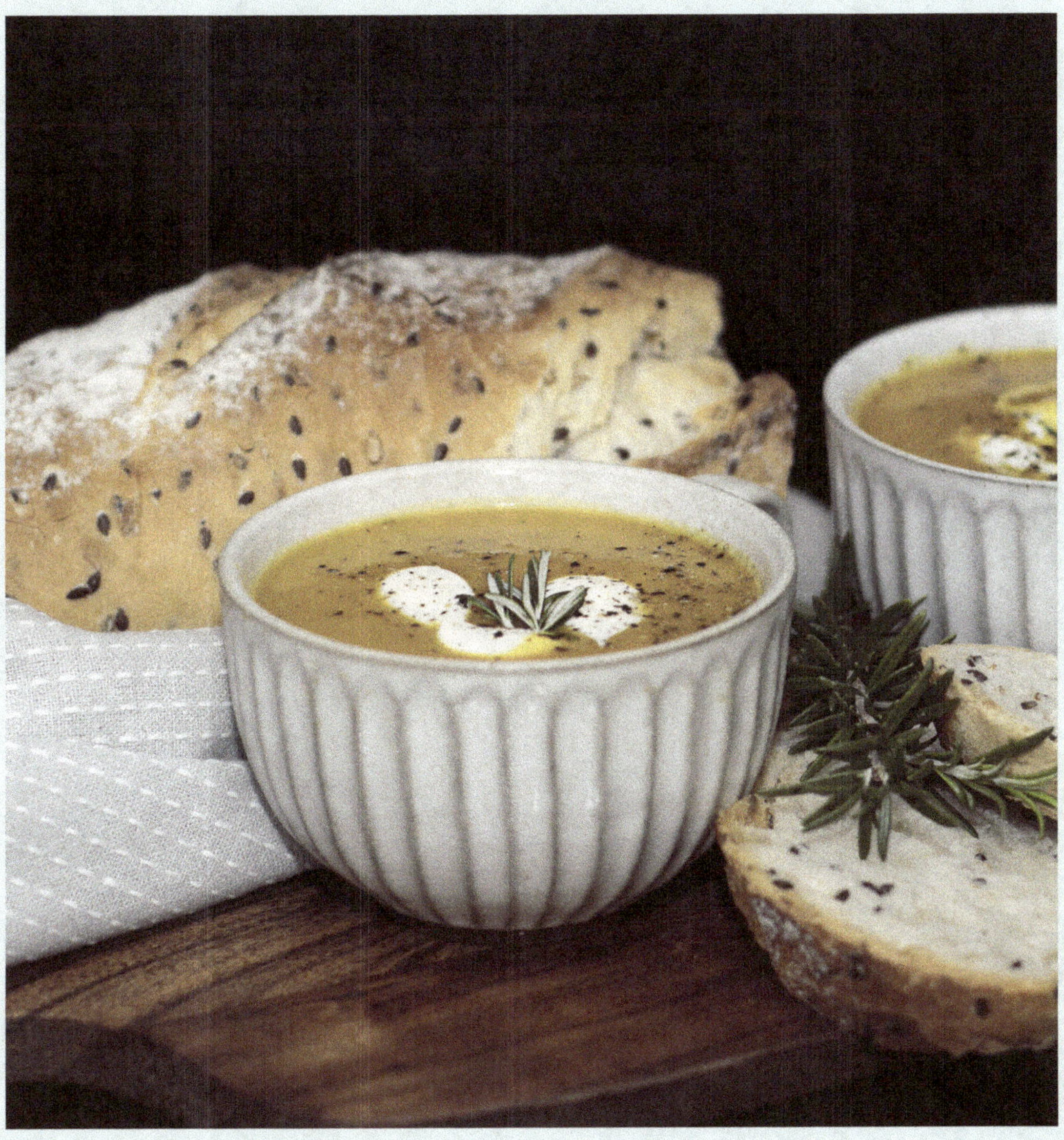

NUTRITIONAL INFORMATION (per serving**):** Calories: 215 kcal | Carbohydrates: 28 g | Protein: 5 g | Fat: 10 g | Saturated Fat: 8 g | Trans Fat: 0 g | Cholesterol: 0 mg | Sodium: 250 mg | Potassium: 728 mg | Fibre: 5 g | Sugar: 4 g | Vitamin A: 10678 IU | Vitamin C: 29 mg | Calcium: 90 mg | Iron: 3 mg

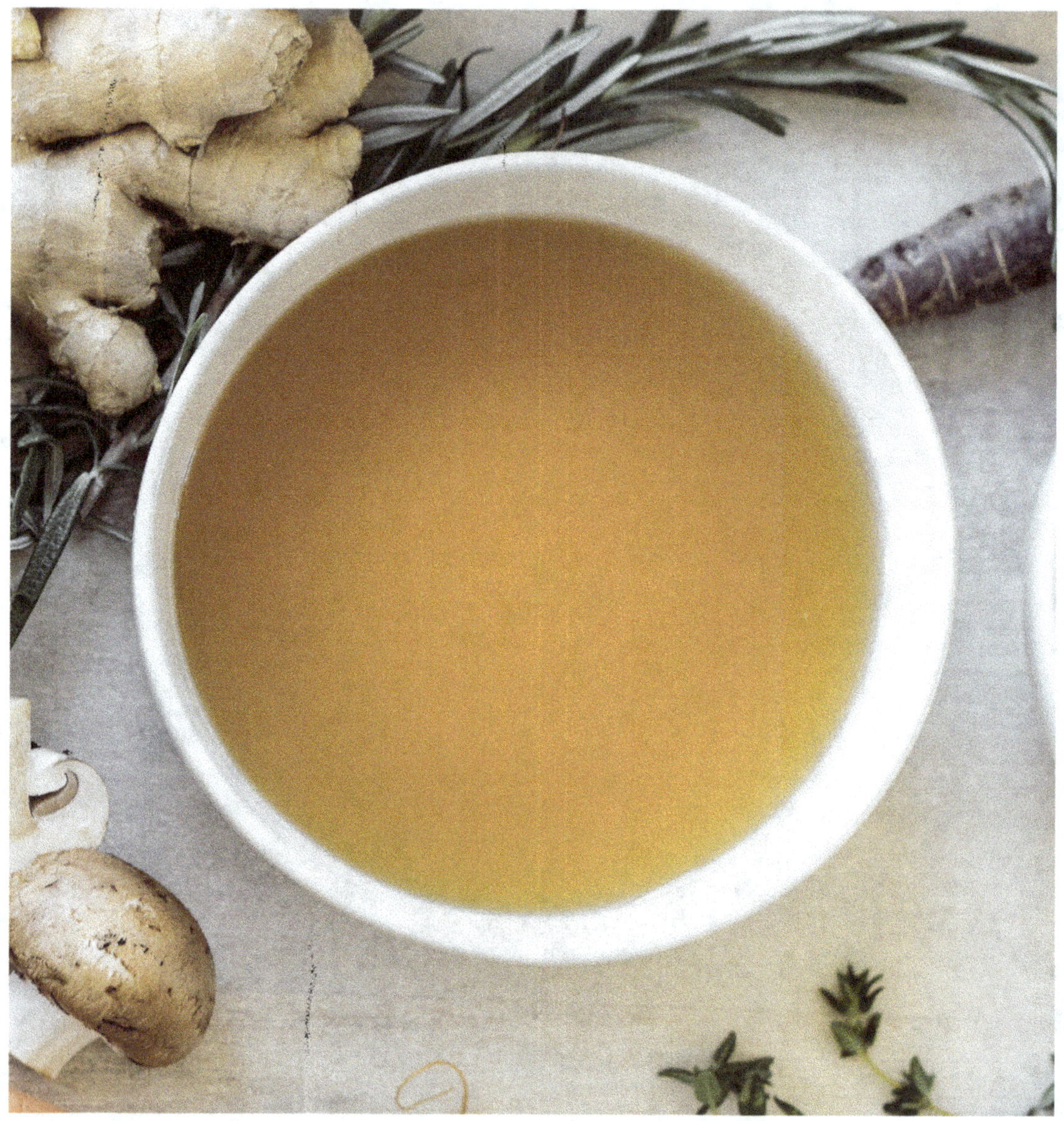

NUTRITIONAL INFORMATION (per serving): Calories: 20 kcal | Carbohydrates: 0 g | Protein: 3 g | Fat: 1 g | Saturated Fat: 0 g | Trans Fat: 0 g | Cholesterol: 0 mg | Sodium: 70 mg | Potassium: 41 mg | Fibre: 0 g | Sugar: 0 g | Vitamin A: 0 IU | Vitamin C: 0 mg | Calcium: 2 mg | Iron: 0 mg

GINGER TURMERIC BONE BROTH
SLOW COOKER RECIPE

PREP TIME 10-15 minutes (preparing bones, measuring and assembling ingredients)

COOKING TIME 24-48 hours on low (slow cooking the bone broth)

TOTAL TIME Approximately 24 hours 10 minutes to 48 hours 15 minutes (including prep and slow cooking time)

INGREDIENTS

Bones for broth (such as chicken or beef)

3-4 litres water

2 tbsp grated ginger

2 tsp turmeric

Pink salt, to taste

METHOD

Place bones, water, grated ginger, turmeric, and pink salt into a slow cooker.

Cook on low heat for 12-24 hours, allowing the flavours to develop and the nutrients to be extracted from the bones.

After the desired cooking time, strain the broth to remove any solids.

The ginger turmeric bone broth is now ready to be used in various recipes or enjoyed on its own for its gut-healing properties.

NOTE: Both of these recipes are designed to support gut health and are packed with nourishing ingredients. The slow cooker method allows for convenient and hands-off preparation. Enjoy the comforting and healing benefits of these delicious soups and broths.

SERVING: The number of servings will depend on the size of your slow cooker and the amount of water used. Generally, a 3- to 4-litre batch of bone broth could yield around 8-12 cups of broth, which would translate to approximately 8-12 servings (1 cup per serving).

CHICKEN CARCASS BROTH
SLOW COOKER RECIPE

PREP TIME 15-20 minutes (preparing ingredients and assembling)

COOKING TIME 12-24 hours on low (slow cooking the broth)

TOTAL TIME Approximately 12 hours 15 minutes to 24 hours 20 minutes (including prep and slow cooking time)

INGREDIENTS

1 bay leaf

2 carrots, peeled and cut in half

2 celery sticks, cut in half

4 garlic cloves, smashed open or cut in half

3-inch piece of fresh ginger

1 white onion, quartered

1/2 tsp whole black peppercorns

2 tsp sea salt

1 tbsp ground turmeric

2 tbsp apple cider vinegar

Enough filtered water to fill the pot

METHOD

In a slow cooker, add chicken carcass, bay leaf, carrots, celery sticks, garlic cloves, ginger, onion, black peppercorns, sea salt, turmeric, and apple cider vinegar. Add enough filtered water to cover the ingredients, about 1/2 inch from the top of the pot.

Cover the slow cooker and set it to low heat. Let it cook for 12-24 hours, or overnight.

Strain the broth through a fine mesh strainer or cheese cloth, discarding all the solids.

You can use the chicken broth as a base for soups or pour it into mason jars to enjoy throughout the week. Allow the broth to come to room temperature before refrigerating.

The broth can be stored in mason jars in the refrigerator for up to 5 days or frozen for up to 2 months.

NOTE: This nourishing chicken carcass broth is rich in flavour and nutrients. It serves as an excellent base for soups or can be consumed on its own for its healing properties. If using for nose tube feeding, ensure proper preparation and handling according to specific medical guidelines

SERVING: The number of servings will depend on the size of your slow cooker and the amount of water used. Generally, a batch of chicken carcass broth could yield around 8-12 cups of broth, which would translate to approximately 8-12 servings (1 cup per serving).

NUTRITIONAL INFORMATION (per serving): Calories: 19 kcal | Carbohydrates: 4 g | Protein: 1 g | Fat: 0 g | Saturated Fat: 0 g | Trans Fat: 0 g | Cholesterol: 0 mg | Sodium: 487 mg | Potassium: 100 mg | Fibre: 1 g | Sugar: 1 g | Vitamin A: 2053 IU | Vitamin C: 3 mg | Calcium: 29 mg | Iron: 1 mg

YOGURT DROPS

PREP TIME 10-15 minutes (preparing igredients and assembling)

COOKING TIME 2-4 hours (freezing time for the drops) |

TOTAL TIME Approximately 2 hours 10 minutes to 4 hours 15 minutes (including prep and freezing time)

INGREDIENTS

1 cup Greek yogurt

1/2 cup pear (30 g)[Use tinned pear or fresh soft pear with the skin removed]

1/2 cup raspberries (25 g)

METHOD

In a blender, combie 1/4 cup Greek yogurt with pear and/or raspberry to make a smooth puree.

Gently stir the puree into the remaining 3/4 cup of Greek yogurt.

Spoon the flavoured yogurt mixture into a piping bag or any small bag with the corner cut off.

Pipe small blobs (buttons) of the flavoured yogurt onto a baking tray or flat plate lined with baking paper or a non-stick reusable liner.

Freeze the yogurt drops until solid, which should take about an hour. Transfer the frozen melts into an airtight container and store them in the freezer until your little one needs a cool yogurt treat.

OTHER FLAVOUR YOGURT MELTS

You can create various flavour combinations by using different fruits and veggies or stirring commercial baby purees through Greek yogurt. Here are some tested options:

1/4 cup Blueberries + 30 g Banana = purple yogurt melts

13 g frozen spinach + 2 tbsp apple sauce = green yogurt melts

TIPS

Use thick yogurt for successful piping of the melts.

Avoid pureeing all the yogurt with the flavourings, as Greek yogurt might lose its thick texture and become too runny to pipe.

Opt for a very small opening when piping the baby yogurt melts, either by cutting a small corner off the bag or using a fine piping tip.

STORAGE

Store the yogurt melts in an airtight container in the freezer for up to 3 months.

Once removed from the freezer, serve them immediately.

SERVING: Around 40-60 drops, depending on their size. The number of servings will depend on the size of the drops and how you portion them.

NUTRITIONAL INFORMATION (per serving): Calories: 53 kcal |
Carbohydrates: 6 g | Protein: 7 g | Fat: 1 g | Saturated Fat: 1 g | Trans Fat: 1 g |
Cholesterol: 3 mg | Sodium: 24 mg | Potassium: 126 mg | Fibre: 1 g | Sugar: 4 g |
Vitamin A: 10 IU | Vitamin C: 3 mg | Calcium: 77 mg | Iron: 1 mg

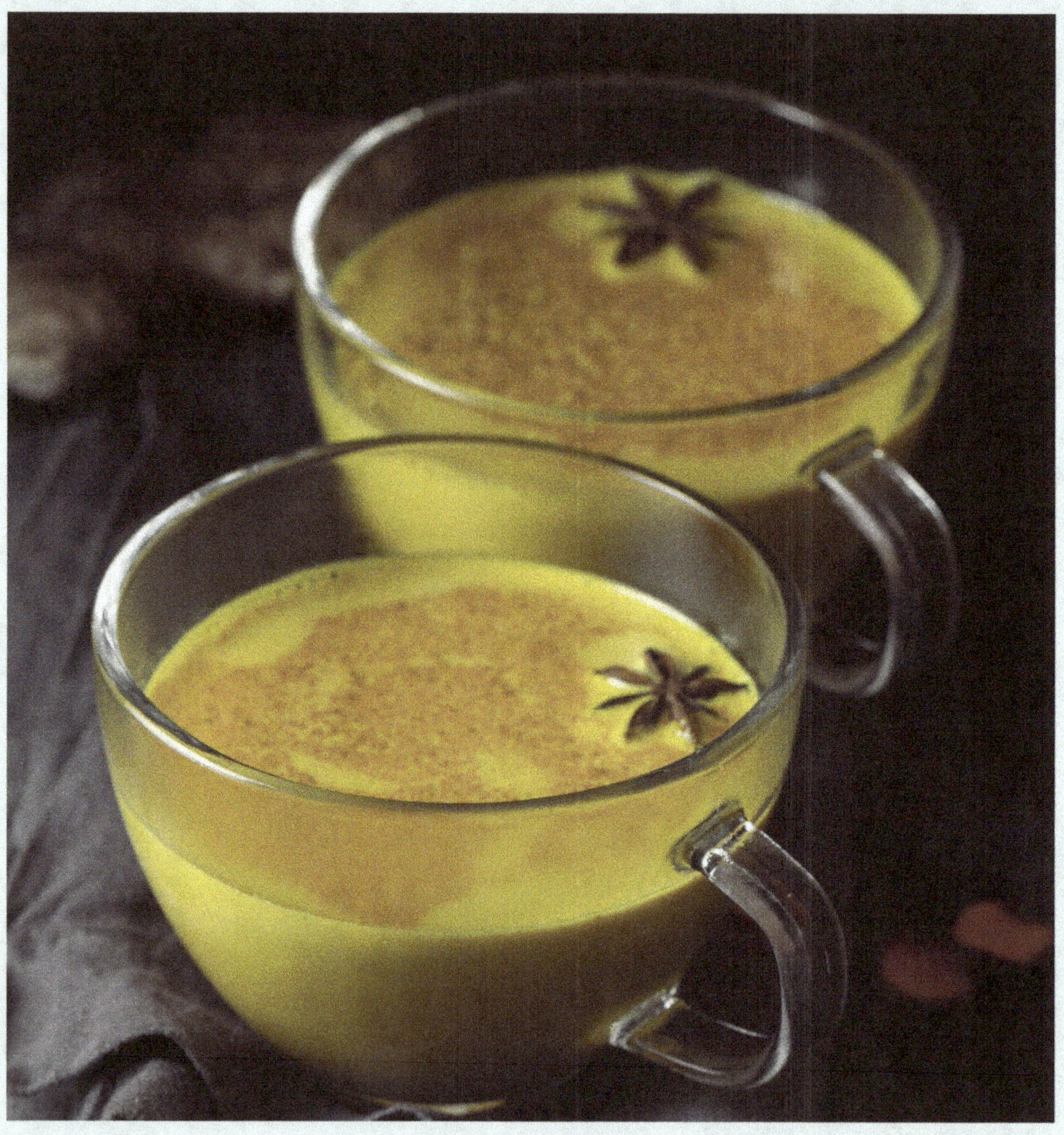

NUTRITIONAL INFORMATION (per serving): Calories: 62 kcal | Carbohydrates: 10 g | Protein: 1 g | Fat: 2 g | Saturated Fat: 0.2 g | Trans Fat: 0 g | Cholesterol: 0 mg | Sodium: 43 mg | Potassium: 80 mg | Fibre: 0 g | Sugar: 8 g | Vitamin D: 0 IU | Calcium: 96 mg | Iron: 1 mg

GOLDEN MILK
ANTI-INFLAMMATORY TURMERIC MILK

PREP TIME 5 minutes (measuring and assembling ingredients)

COOKING TIME 5-7 minutes (heating and simmering the latte)

TOTAL TIME 10-12 minutes

INGREDIENTS

125 mL (1/2 cup) non-dairy milk

1 tsp turmeric

1 tbsp grated ginger or 1/2 tsp ginger powder

1 tsp honey

Pinch of black pepper

BENEFITS

Reducing inflammation

Preventing cell damage and aiding in cell repair

Supporting brain function and improving memory

Boosting the immune system

Improving bone health with vitamin D and calcium

METHOD

In a pot, combine all the ingredients.

Bring the mixture to a boil and then reduce the heat to a simmer.

Simmer for 10 minutes, allowing the flavours to infuse.

Strain the mixture to remove the spices.

The golden milk can be stored in the refrigerator for up to 5 days.

Note: Golden milk, made with the goodness of turmeric, ginger, and other spices, is a nourishing and comforting beverage. Enjoy it warm for its anti-inflammatory properties and numerous health benefits. Feel free to adjust the sweetness and spice levels to suit your taste preferences.

FRUIT PANCAKES

PREP TIME 10-15 minutes (measuring and mixing ingredients) |

COOKING TIME 15-20 minutes (cooking the pancakes)

TOTAL TIME Approximately 25-35 minutes (including prep and cooking time)

INGREDIENTS

1 ½ cups rolled oats (150 g)

½ cup apple puree (150 g)

1 tsp baking powder

1 tsp vanilla extract

½ cup milk (125 mL) or milk substitute

1 tbsp maple syrup (15 mL)

METHOD

In a food processor, pulse the rolled oats until finely ground. If using a blender, you can directly add all the ingredients to it and skip this step.

Add apple puree, baking powder, vanilla extract, milk, and maple syrup to the food processor or blender. Blend until the mixture becomes smooth and thick.

Heat a greased pan over medium heat and drop spoonsful of the batter onto it.

Flip the pancakes when bubbles form and burst on the surface.

Let the pancakes cool slightly before serving.

NOTES:

To avoid quick browning due to high fruit content, cook the pancakes over lower heat for a slightly longer time instead of using high heat.

Both food processors and blenders work well for making the batter. If using a blender, ensure it has a vent to release any pressure that may build up once the raising agents are added.

These pancakes freeze well. Store them in an airtight container and freeze for up to 3 months.

For ingredient substitutions, you can use any dairy-free milk alternative, omit or replace maple syrup with a small amount of honey (for kids over 1 year old), use traditional rolled oats or quick-cook oats, substitute apple puree with a large banana, and replace vanilla with cinnamon for a different flavour.

If you don't have baking powder, you can use ¼ tsp of baking soda instead.

SERVING: Approximately 6–8 medium-sized pancakes, which is roughly 2-3 servings, depending on portion sizes. The number of servings will depend on the size of your pancakes and how many you make with the batter.

NUTRITIONAL INFORMATION (per serving – 1 pancake): Calories: 54 kcal | Carbohydrates: 10 g | Protein: 2 g | Fat: 1 g | Saturated Fat: 1 g | Cholesterol: 1 mg | Sodium: 86 mg | Potassium: 62 mg | Fibre: 1 g | Sugar: 2 g | Vitamin A: 19 IU | Vitamin C: 1 mg | Calcium: 39 mg | Iron: 1 mg

VEGEMITE CHEDDAR CRACKERS

PREP TIME 15-20 minutes (measuring and mixing ingredients, forming and cutting crackers)

COOKING TIME 10-15 minutes (baking the crackers)

TOTAL TIME Approximately 25-35 minutes (including prep and cooking time)

INGREDIENTS

225g sharp cheddar cheese, finely shredded

1 cup all-purpose flour

1 teaspoon salt, plus extra for topping

55g unsalted butter, cubed, at room temperature

2 tablespoons cold whole milk

1 tablespoon Vegemite

METHOD

Preheat the oven to 160°C (325°F) ad line baking sheets with parchment paper.

In a food processor or using a standard mixer fitted with a paddle attachment, combine the chese, flour, and salt. Pulse several times until well mixed.

Add the butter and Vegemite to the mixture and pulse a few more times until the dough becomes dry and crumbly.

Pour in the cold milk and pulse several more times. Test the dough by pressing it between two fingers to see if it holds together. If not, pulse a few more times and test again.

Transfer the dough onto a lightly floured surface and divide it into two equal pieces. Roll each piece into a very thin rectangle.

Using a pastry wheel or knife, slice the dough into 1-inch squares. Use the flat end of a skewer to poke a hole all the way through each cracker.

Arrange the squares on the prepared baking sheets and sprinkle with extra salt.

Bake for 17-20 minutes, or until the edges turn a deep golden brown and the crackers puff slightly. Allow them to cool before enjoying.

These crackers will keep for up to 1 week in a sealed container at room temperature. Enjoy!

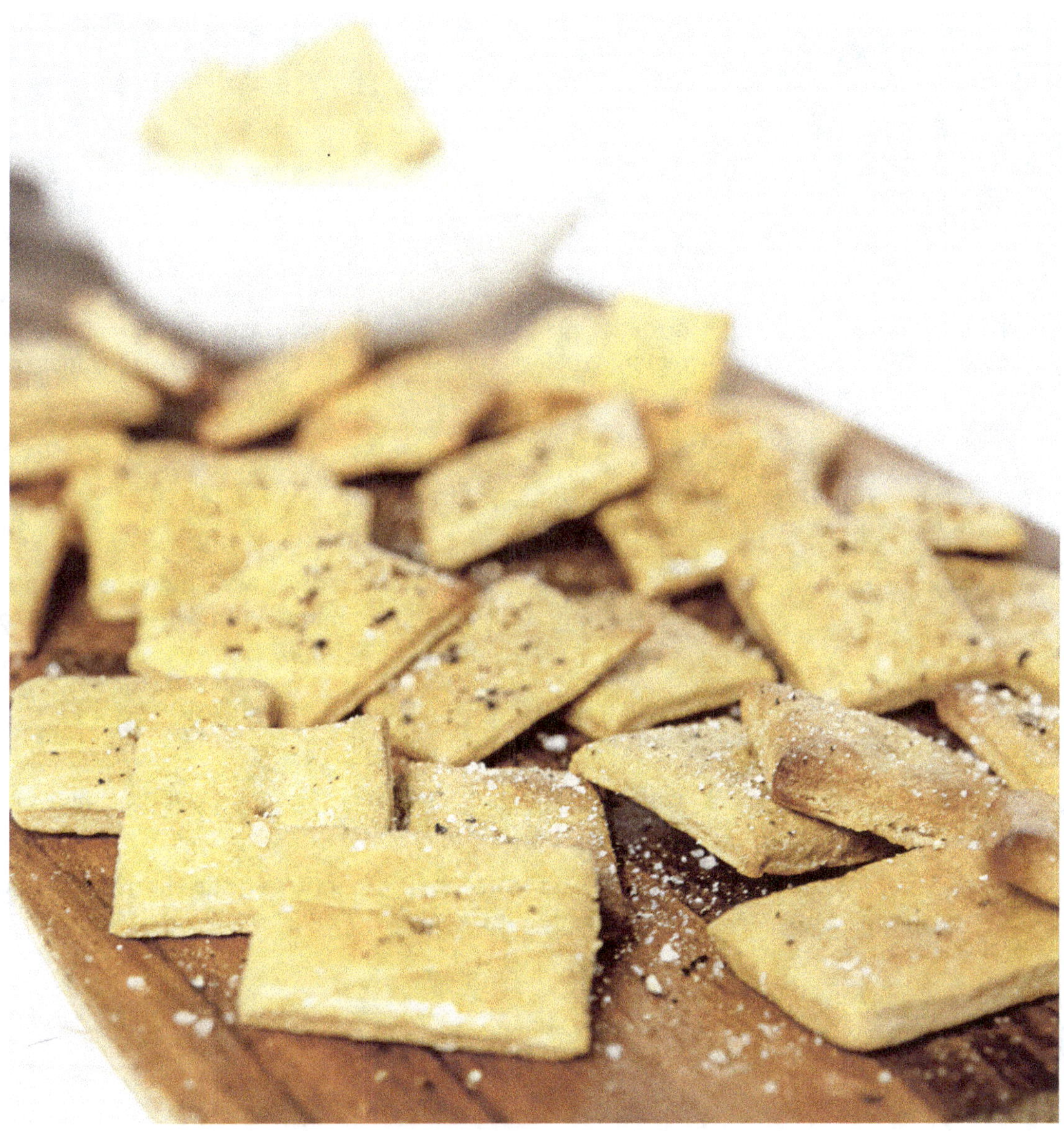

NUTRITIONAL INFORMATION for the Whole Recipe: Calories: 1498 kcal | Carbohydrates: 208 g | Protein: 18 g | Fat: 71 g | Saturated Fat: 47 g | Trans Fat: 0 g | Cholesterol: 0 mg | Sodium: 602 mg | Potassium: 458 mg | Fibre: 8 g | Sugar: 68 g | Vitamin A: 256 IU | Vitamin C: 0 mg | Calcium: 94 mg | Iron: 7 mg

NO-BAKE WEETABIX SLICE

PREP TIME 15-20 minutes (measuring and processing ingredients, assembling) |

COOKING TIME No cooking required (being a no-bake recipe)

TOTAL TIME Approximately 15-20 minutes (including prep time)

INGREDIENTS

5 Weetabix (75 g)

1 cup pitted dates

1/2 cup sunflower seeds

1/2 cup desiccated coconut

4 tbsp cocoa

2 tbsp honey

2 tbsp water

40 g dark chocolate (optional)

METHOD

In a food processor, blend the first seven ingredients until they form a ball. It may take 3-5 minutes. If needed, add 1-2 tbsp of water while blending.

Line a loaf tin with baking paper while the food processor is running.

If using dark chocolate, melt it using a double boiler or short bursts in the microwave.

Press the mixture into the loaf tin and add the melted chocolate on top (optional).

Refrigerate for 2 hours.

Slice and enjoy!

NOTES:

Store the slice in the refrigerator for 3-5 days, or freeze for longer storage.

Be patient with the food processor; the mixture might take time to come together.

If the mixture doesn't combine well, add 1-2 tbsp of water.

Soak dates in warm water or microwave with a splash of water if needed.

Regular dried dates or softer Medjool dates can be used.

Substitute ingredients as desired (generic cereal, different nuts or seeds, raisins, sultanas, coconut).

Honey can be replaced with rice malt syrup or maple syrup.

For dairy-free, use dairy-free dark chocolate or skip the chocolate layer.

For wheat and gluten-free, use gluten-free Weetabix.

SERVING: Around 12-16 small slices, which is roughly 6-8 servings, depending on portion sizes. The number of servings will depend on the size of the slices you cut.

NUTRITIONAL INFORMATION (per serving): Calories: 95 kcal | Carbohydrates: 13 g | Protein: 2 g | Fat: 5 g | Saturated Fat: 2 g | Cholesterol: 1 mg | Sodium: 3 mg | Potassium: 140 mg | Fibre: 2 g | Sugar: 9 g | Vitamin C: 1 mg | Calcium: 11 mg | Iron: 1 mg

GOLDEN TURMERIC OATMEAL

PREP TIME 5 minutes (measuring and mixing ingredients)

COOKING TIME 10-15 minutes (cooking the oatmeal)

TOTAL TIME Approximately 15-20 minutes (including prep and cooking time)

INGREDIENTS

1/2 cup rolled oats

1 1/4 cups milk (use your favourite, almond or oat milk for a vegan option)

1/4 tsp powdered turmeric

1/4 tsp cinnamon

1/4 tsp powdered ginger

Pinch of black pepper

Maple syrup or date paste, to taste

METHOD

In a saucepan, add all the ingredients, except the sweetener, and gently bring the mixture to a boil.

Reduce the heat to a simmer and continue to cook for about 10 minutes, stirring frequently, until the mixture has thickened.

Add your preferred sweetener to taste, then pour the oatmeal into a bowl.

Add your favourite toppings, if desired.

NOTES:

Adjust the amount of milk according to your desired consistency.

Feel free to customize your toppings with fruits, nuts, or seeds.

For a nut-free version, use sunflower seeds or other seeds instead of cashews

SERVING: Approximately 1 serving of golden turmeric oatmeal.

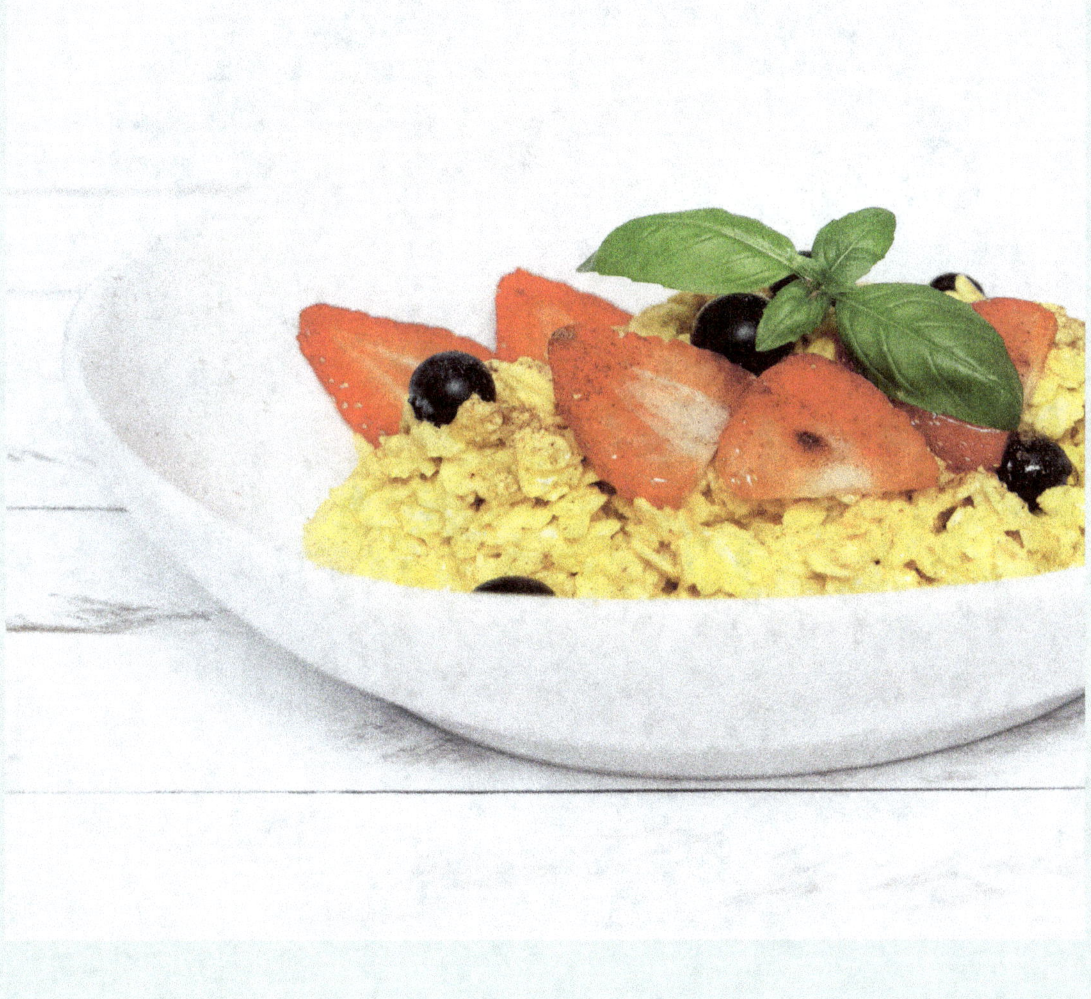

NUTRITIONAL INFORMATION (per serving): Calories: About 300–350 kcal | Carbohydrates: Approximately 50–60 g | Protein: About 10–12 g | Fat: Around 5–7 g | Sodium: Varies based on ingredients and added salt | Fibre: Roughly 6–8 g

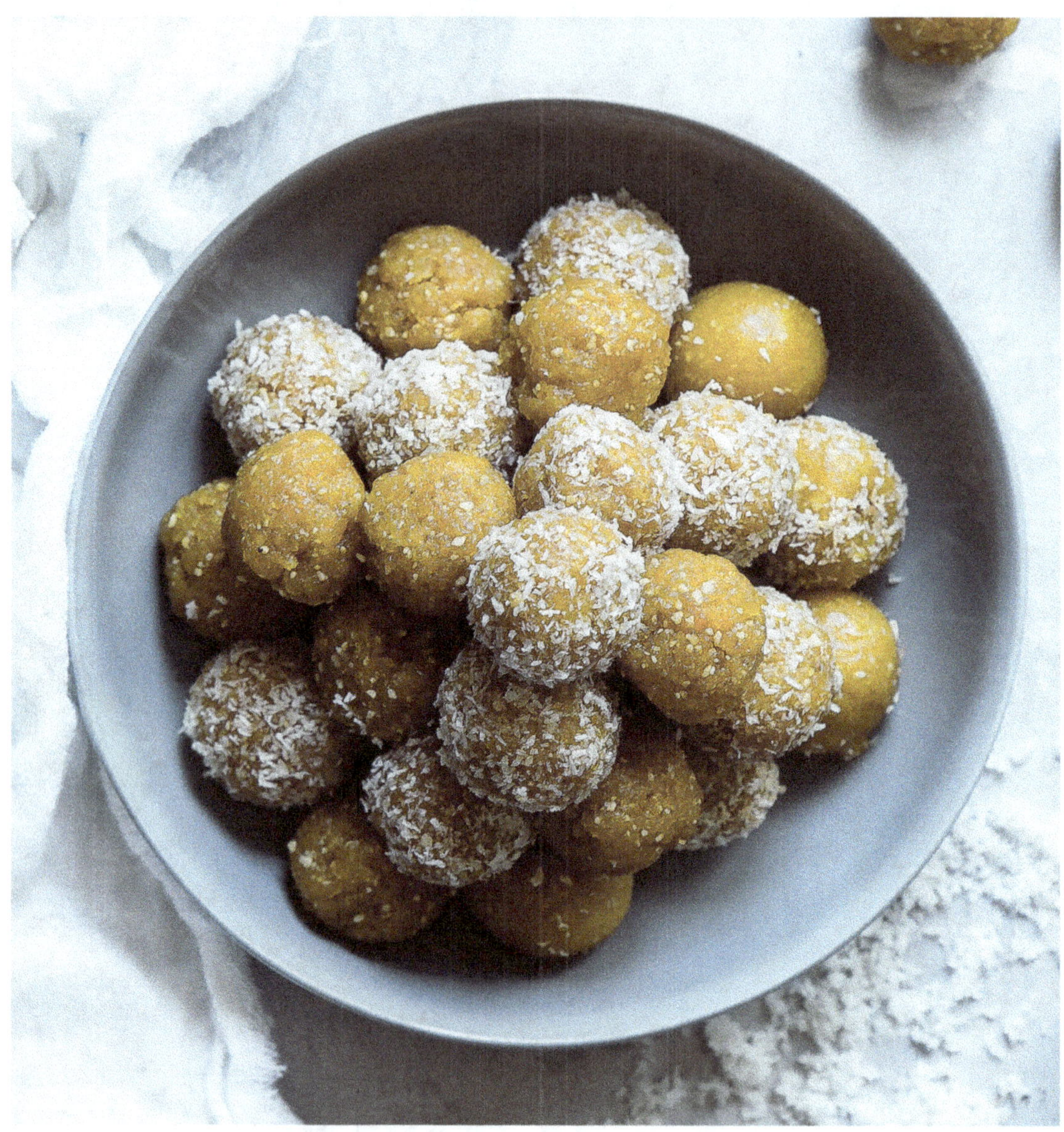

NUTRITIONAL INFORMATION: Serving Size: 1 slice | Calories: 55 kcal | Total Fat: 1 g | Saturated Fat: 0 g | Trans Fat: 0 g | Unsaturated Fat: 1 g | Cholesterol: 0 mg | Sodium: 34 mg | Carbohydrates: 11 g | Fibre: 1 g | Sugar: 5 g | Protein: 1 g

APRICOT ENERGY BALLS

PREP TIME 15-20 minutes (measuring and processing ingredients, shaping the balls)

COOKING TIME No cooking required

TOTAL TIME Approximately 15-20 minutes (including prep time)

INGREDIENTS

4 Weet-Bix, Weetabix, or Wheat Biscuits

1 cup unsalted roasted cashews

1 cup dried apricots

Water

METHOD

In a food processor, blitz the ingredients until they are finely ground.

Slowly add water (1-2 tbsp) until the mixture comes together into a ball.

Line a loaf tin with baking paper and press the mixture into it, making it around 2-cm thick at the base.

Chill the mixture in the refrigerator for 2 hours.

Slice the chilled mixture into serving portions. and store in the refrigerator or freezer.

NOTES:

Roasted cashews are preferred, but unroasted will also work.

If your food processor is not very powerful, soak the dried apricots in warm water, drain well before making the recipe.

You can shape the mixture into balls instead of making a slice.

For a nut-free version, substitute cashews with sunflower seeds.

Those with gluten sensitivity can use gluten-free Weetabix for a wheat and gluten-free alternative.

VEGEMITE PASTA

A RECIPE BY DAVID LOVETT, AUTHOR OF THE "BIG & LITTLE COOKBOOK."

PREP TIME 5 minutes (melting butter and preparing Vegemite)

COOKING TIME 10-15 minutes (cooking the pasta)

TOTAL TIME Approximately 15-20 minutes (including prep and cooking time)

INGREDIENTS

1 tbsp melted butter

Heaped tbsp of Vegemite

Pasta (any shape)

METHOD

In a pan over medium heat, melt 1 tbsp of butter gently.

Add 2 tbsp of Vegemite and stir until it melts together. Turn off the heat.

Cook pasta per the instructions.

Drain the pasta, but remember to keep 2 tbsp of pasta water.

Combine the pasta and pasta water with the butter and Vegemite mixture. Mix everything together well. You can also add some cheese, such as parmesan, for extra flavour.

NOTE: Feel free to adjust the amount of Vegemite to suit your taste preferences. Enjoy!

SERVING: The number of servings will depend on the amount of pasta you cook. This recipe provides the flavouring for the pasta, and you can adjust the quantities based on the number of servings you need. It's typically suitable for 2-4 servings of pasta.

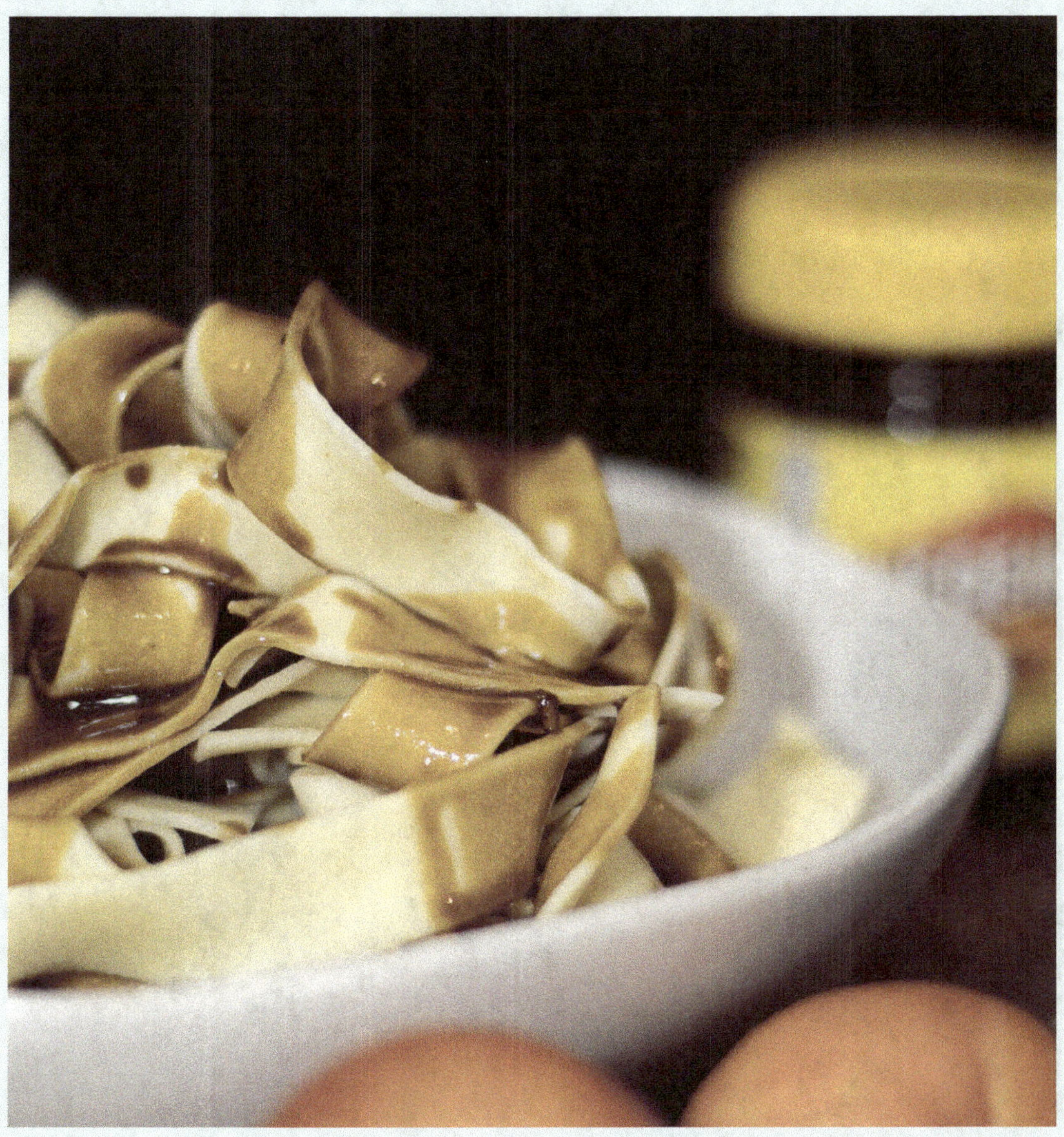

NUTRITIONAL INFORMATION: Calories: 125 kcal | Carbohydrates: 20 g | Protein: 4 g | Fat: 3 g | Saturated Fat: 2 g | Trans Fat: 0 g | Cholesterol: 8 mg | Sodium: 95 mg | Potassium: 40 mg | Fibre: 1 g | Sugar: 1 g | Vitamin A: 98 IU | Vitamin C: 0 mg | Calcium: 4 mg | Iron: 1 mg

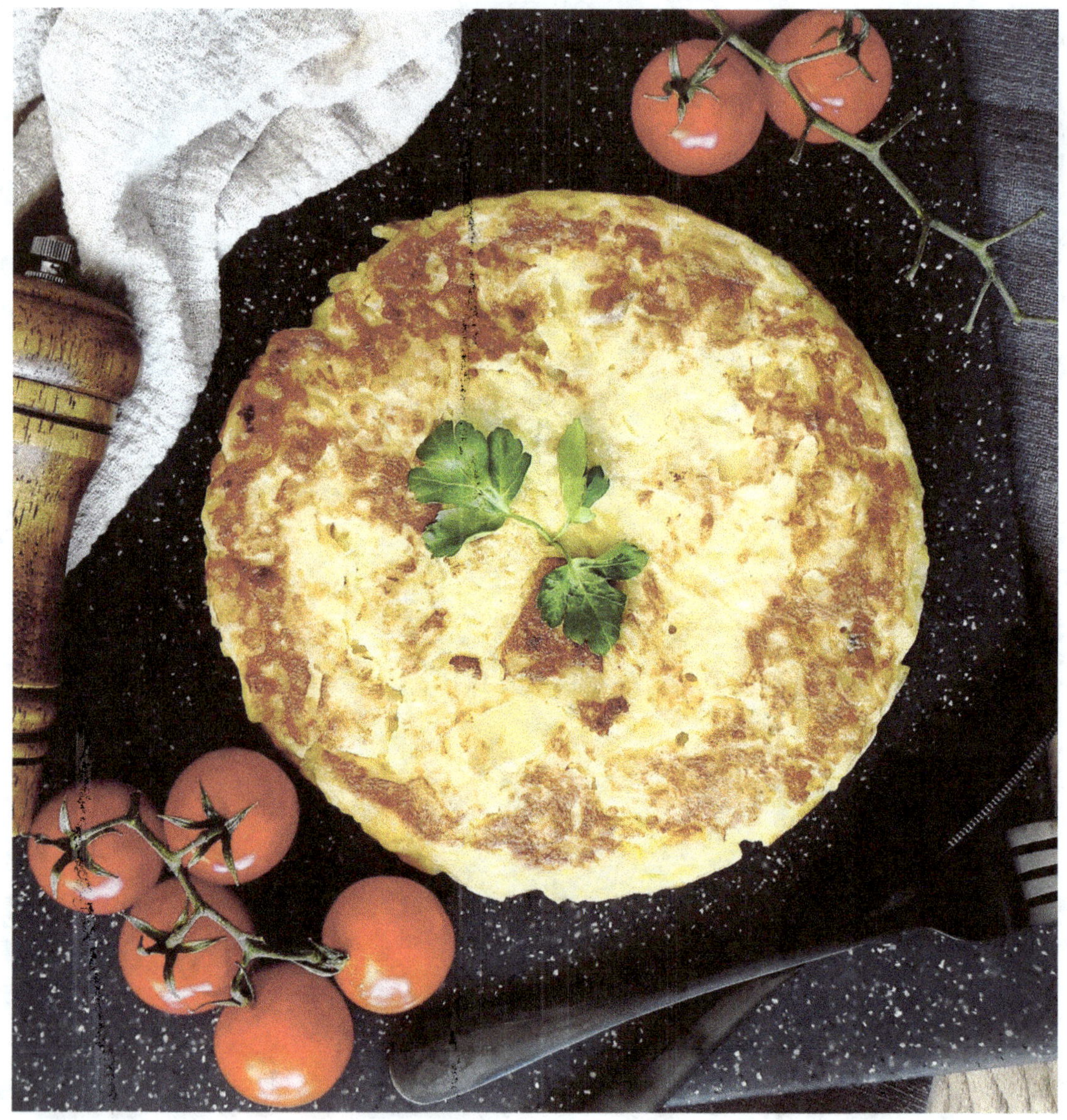

NUTRITIONAL INFORMATION (per serving): Calories: 330 kcal | Protein: 26.8 g | Fat: 47.8 g | Net Carbs: 1.5 g | Fibre: 6.6 g

CHEESE OMELETTE

PREP TIME 5-7 minutes (cracking eggs, grating cheese, slicing vegetables)

COOKING TIME 5-7 minutes (cooking the omelette)

TOTAL TIME Approximately 10-14 minutes (including prep and cooking time)

INGREDIENTS

2 large eggs

Salt and pepper

50 g cheddar cheese, grated

1 tbsp butter

5 cherry tomatoes (optional)

1/2 medium avocado (optional)

Bacon (optional, for children going through the "salt phase")

METHOD

Crack eggs into a bowl and whisk to combine. Season with salt and pepper.

In a small frying pan, melt butter over medium heat. Pour in the whisked eggs and swirl the pan until the eggs cover the base of the frying pan evenly. Scatter grated cheese on one side of the eggs.

Reduce the heat to medium-low and cook the omelette for about 3 minutes, or until the eggs start to set and the cheese melts.

Using a spatula, carefully fold the omelette in half. Transfer it to a plate and serve it hot, optionally with cherry tomatoes and avocado on the side. For children going through the "salt phase," you can also add bacon to the omelette.

NOTE: This recipe can be customised by adding or omitting optional ingredients based on personal preferences and dietary needs. Enjoy!

SERVING: This recipe is typically for a single serving omelette. However, you can easily adjust the quantities to make more servings if needed.

ONE-PAN CREAMY CHICKEN AND MUSHROOM SKILLET

PREP TIME 15-20 minutes (preparing ingredients and assembling)

COOKING TIME 25-30 minutes (cooking the dish) |

TOTAL TIME Approximately 40-50 minutes (including prep and cooking time)

INGREDIENTS

Juice of 1/2 lemon

1 garlic clove, minced

1/2 tsp chopped lemon thyme leaves

1/2 tsp chopped rosemary leaves

Salt and pepper

4 boneless chicken thighs, skin on

1 tbsp olive oil

1 diced onion

125 g sliced mushrooms

1/2 cup full-fat sour cream

1/2 tsp ground nutmeg

120 g baby spinach

METHOD

In a large bowl, combine lemon juice, minced garlic, chopped lemon thyme, and rosemary leaves. Season with salt and pepper. Add chicken thighs, skin side up, and coat them with the marinade. Set the chicken aside for at least 5 minutes or marinate overnight for more flavour.

In a frying pan, heat olive oil over medium heat. Add the chicken thighs, skin side down, and brown them for 5-7 minutes. Flip the chicken over and cook for another 5-7 minutes. Transfer the chicken to a plate and set it aside.

In the same pan, add the diced onion and cook for 2-3 minutes until translucent. Add the sliced mushrooms and cook for an additional 5 minutes.

Stir in sour cream and ground nutmeg, combining well. Add baby spinach and return the chicken thighs to the pan, skin side up. Cook for another 10 minutes or until the sauce thickens nicely, and the chicken is cooked through.

Optionally, you can serve this dish with pasta or fresh bread.

SERVING: 2-3 servings, depending on portion sizes and appetites.

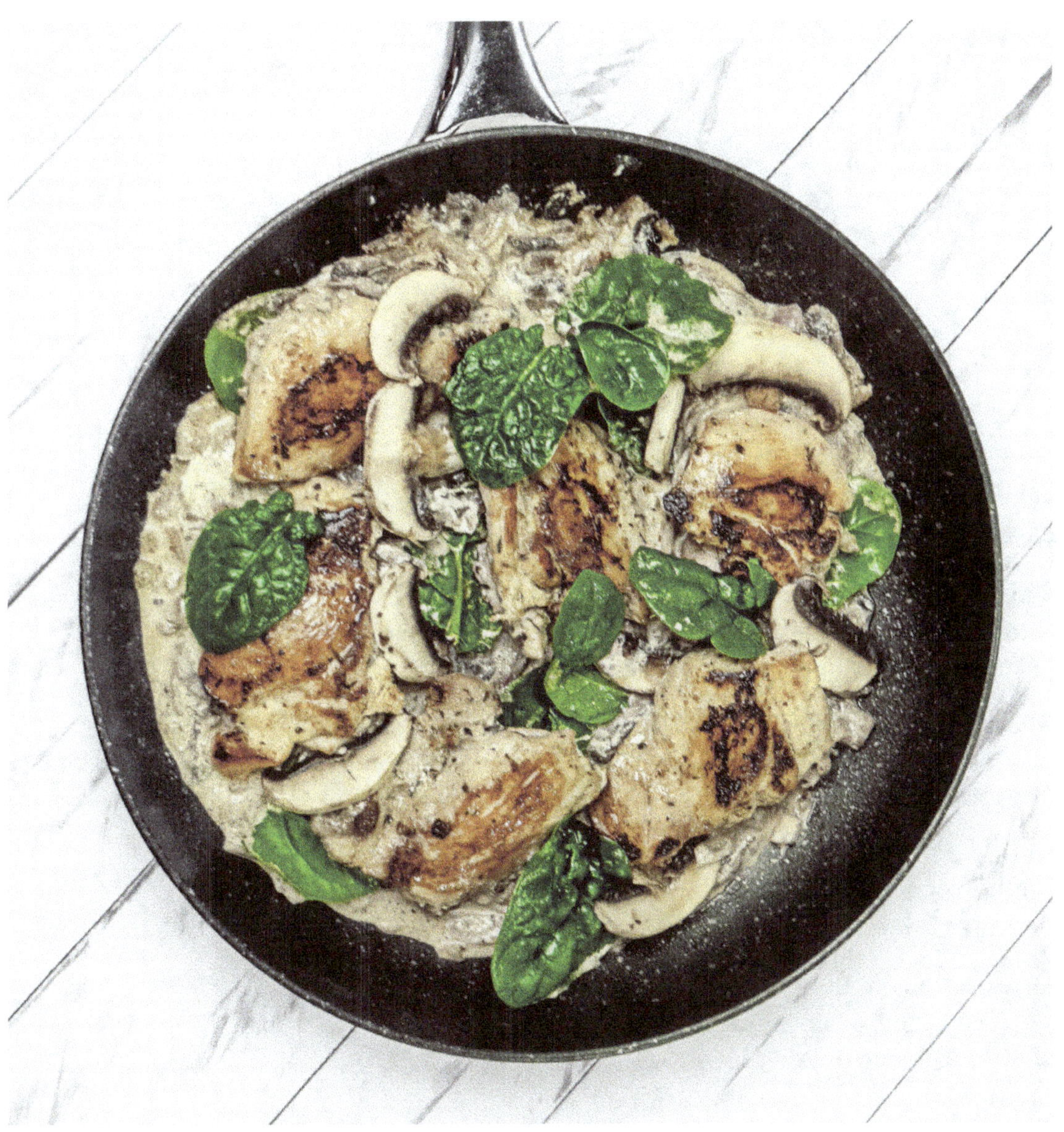

NUTRITIONAL INFORMATION for the Whole Recipe: Calories: 1052 kcal | Carbohydrates: 15 g | Protein: 72 g | Fat: 77 g | Saturated Fat: 26 g | Trans Fat: 0 g | Cholesterol: 319 mg | Sodium: 530 mg | Potassium: 1368 mg | Fibre: 3 g | Sugar: 5 g | Vitamin A: 5140 IU | Vitamin C: 15 mg | Calcium: 172 mg | Iron: 5 mg

NUTRIENT-PACKED POWER BITES: HIGH-CALORIE SNACKS FOR NOURISHMENT

NUT BUTTER AND WHOLE GRAIN CRACKERS

SERVING SIZE: 2 tbsp of nut butter with 4 whole grain crackers
CALORIES: Approximately 250-300 calories per serving

CHEESE AND FRUIT PLATE

SERVING SIZE: 1 ounce of cheese (28 g) with a small apple or pear
CALORIES: Approximately 150-200 calories per serving

GREEK YOGURT WITH HONEY AND NUTS

SERVING SIZE: 1 cup of Greek yogurt (240 g) with 1 tbsp of honey and 1 tbsp of chopped nuts
CALORIES: Approximately 300-350 calories per serving

AVOCADO TOAST ON WHOLE GRAIN BREAD

SERVING SIZE: ½ ripe avocado (about 100 g) on 2 slices of whole grain bread
CALORIES: Approximately 250-300 calories per serving

TRAIL MIX

SERVING SIZE: 1/4 cup of trail mix (about 30 g)
CALORIES: Approximately 150-200 calories per serving

PEANUT BUTTER AND BANANA SMOOTHIE

SERVING SIZE: 1 cup of whole milk, 1 banana, and 2 tbsp of peanut butter blended together
CALORIES: Approximately 300-350 calories per serving

HOMEMADE ENERGY BITES

SERVING SIZE: 2 energy bites (about 40 g)
CALORIES: Approximately 200-250 calories per serving

HUMMUS WITH WHOLE GRAIN PITA BREAD

SERVING SIZE: 1/2 cup of hummus with 2 whole grain pita bread (about 50 g each)
CALORIES: Approximately 250-300 calories per serving

CHEESE QUESADILLA

SERVING SIZE: 1 whole grain tortilla (about 50 g) filled with 1/2 cup of shredded cheese
CALORIES: Approximately 250-300 calories per serving

MASHED AVOCADO ON RICE CAKES

SERVING SIZE: 1 mashed avocado (about 100 g) spread on 2 rice cakes
CALORIES: Approximately 200-250 calories per serving

* Please note that the calorie content may vary based on the specific brands and ingredients used.

MOVING FORWARD

This chapter covers embracing play, post-treatment wellness after treatment, and navigating chemo brain (brain fog).

NAVIGATING POST-TREATMENT CHALLENGES

After completing cancer treatment, children enter a phase known as "survivorship." Clinically, cancer survivorship begins at diagnosis itself but rather than simply focusing on cancer treatment and management (as done in the past), it extends to patients' experience and life after finishing treatment and remaining cancer free. This period can be both a joyous milestone and a time of adjustment, as children and their families transition back to a more normal routine. It is essential to recognize that the post-cancer phase throws its unique challenges and opportunities for growth. Here is some information on children after cancer treatment:

PHYSICAL HEALTH: Children may experience a myriad of physical health milestones after cancer treatment. While some may quickly regain their strength and energy, others may face lingering side effects or long-term health issues. Thus, regular medical check-ups and follow-ups are vital to monitor their health and address any concerns promptly.

EMOTIONAL WELL-BEING: The emotional impact of surviving cancer can vary from child to child. While some may feel relieved and happy, others may experience anxiety, fear, or uncertainty about their future. Providing emotional support, encouraging open communication, and seeking professional counselling if needed can assist in their emotional well-being.

TRANSITION TO SCHOOL AND SOCIAL LIFE: Returning to school and social activities is an essential part of resuming a normal life after cancer treatment. Some children may need support to reintegrate into school and cope with changes in friendships or social dynamics.

NUTRITION AND LIFESTYLE: After cancer treatment, maintaining a healthy lifestyle, including balanced nutrition and regular physical activity, becomes all the more important. Parents and caregivers should encourage healthy eating habits and age-appropriate physical activities to support their child's overall well-being.

LATE EFFECTS AND SURVIVORSHIP CLINICS: Some children may experience late effects of cancer treatment, which can manifest months or years after treatment completion. Hence, regular visits to survivorship clinics can help monitor and manage these late effects to ensure optimal long-term health outcomes.

CELEBRATING MILESTONES AND RESILIENCE: Celebrating milestones, big and small, can provide a sense of accomplishment and boost morale. Emphasizing the child's resilience and strength in overcoming cancer can foster a positive self-image and promote coping skills for future challenges.

SUPPORTIVE CARE AND ADVOCACY: Access to supportive care services and resources is essential for the child's continued well-being. Parents and caregivers play a vital role in advocating for their child's needs and ensuring they receive the necessary support throughout their survivorship journey.

QUALITY OF LIFE: Emphasizing the child's quality of life is paramount. Balancing medical follow-ups with age-appropriate activities, hobbies, and social interactions can contribute to a well-rounded and fulfilling life.

FUTURE HEALTH MONITORING: Monitoring the child's health, both physical and emotional, should be an ongoing priority. Regular communication with the healthcare team and open dialogues with the child can aid in detecting any emerging health concerns.

GRATITUDE AND HOPE: The post-cancer phase is an opportunity to express gratitude for the successful treatment and to embrace hope for a bright and promising future. With the right support and care, children can move forward with confidence and optimism, leaving cancer behind them as they embark on new adventures.

Overall, the post-treatment journey of children is marked by resilience, growth, and a renewed appreciation for life. Nurturing their physical health, emotional well-being, and social connections is essential in helping them thrive as cancer survivors.

After Jake's treatment, we noticed that he had difficulty sitting still for extended periods; he preferred being active and on the move. On days when he felt a bit lethargic or had some downtime, he tended to eat less and even made comments about his body weight, expressing concerns about looking "fat." It was heart-wrenching for us to hear, especially because we could see that he was finally looking healthier after his treatment. This struggle with body image appeared to be a common hurdle among other children and teens who had experienced cancer treatment. Many of them had become accustomed to seeing themselves as skin and bones, and adjusting to a healthier physique could be mentally challenging. What brought about a positive change for Jake was a simple but powerful moment during a visit to his doctor. The doctor measured his height and casually mentioned that Jake was on track to be tall and slender. In that moment, something shifted for Jake. He looked up and asked, "So I'm not going to be fat?" It was like a light bulb went off in his mind. The doctor's comment seemed to provide him with reassurance and helped dispel his fear of gaining weight. From that point forward, we noticed a positive shift in Jake's behaviour. He started having more substantial meals and allowed himself proper downtime without feeling guilty. The doctor's affirmation had somehow empowered him to embrace a healthier self-image.

As parents, witnessing this transformation reinforced the significance of creating a supportive and understanding environment for children during and after cancer treatment, highlighting the implication of addressing their emotional well-being and body image concerns, along with their physical health. Every child's journey is unique, and offering compassion, patience, and encouragement can play a key role in helping them navigate through these challenging times with a positive outlook.

As Jake's treatment neared its end, he started experiencing deep feelings of depression, which was understandable given all that he had been through. It puzzled us why these emotions surfaced at this decisive time when we thought he would be feeling relief. He started losing interest in eating and engaging in activities outside the house, and we were concerned about his well-being. The turning point came unexpectedly when Jake's NG tube got accidentally pulled out during playtime with his sister. We braced ourselves for a breakdown, but something different happened this time. After talking with Jake about the incident, we made a pivotal decision. Considering he was nearing the end of his treatment, we agreed to leave the NG tube out if he could make an effort to eat more. To our surprise, it was like witnessing a shining star. Jake embraced the opportunity and started eating more regularly. He regained his enthusiasm for life, playing with his sisters and the neighbouring boys. It was as if removing the NG tube had lifted a weight off his shoulders, and he even remarked that now he could wear a hat and not feel sick anymore.

Reflecting on the experience, we realized that the NG tube had unwittingly affected Jake's self-perception. The tube had become a constant reminder of his illness, and by removing it, he felt liberated and more like himself again. It was a profound realization for us as parents, and we couldn't be more grateful for the peace of mind the NG tube had provided throughout his treatment. Indeed, the NG tube had been a lifeline during challenging times when Jake needed it most, ensuring he received his medicine and nourishment even when he lacked the strength to eat. However, its presence also exerted an unexpected impact on Jake's self-image. We learned that acknowledging and understanding a child's perspective during treatment can significantly influence their emotional well-being and recovery. In the end, the NG tube had played a crucial role in Jake's journey, and while we had never anticipated its effect on his self-esteem, we were relieved that its removal brought him newfound joy and the ability to embrace life as he moved forward beyond cancer treatment.

After completing his cancer treatment, there was a period where we continued to have follow-up appointments at the hospital. Surprisingly, Jake would express his desire to have a sleepover at the hospital. One might think that he had enough of hospital stays, but the reality was different. Hospital visits had become such a significant part of his life since he was just 6 years old, and he couldn't remember much before that time. For him, the hospital was a familiar and somewhat comforting place. Perhaps, he needed a transition phase after treatment, and returning to the hospital for check-ups allowed him to slowly adjust to life beyond cancer treatment. The hospital had become a symbol of hope and care during his challenging journey, and a part of him wanted to hold onto that sense of security a little longer.

Despite some definite hard times during our hospital visits, we also tried to make it fun and enjoyable for Jake. We had lunch dates where we would watch Ellen or MasterChef while having a meal together. We played video games together, and he also spent time with a couple of boys on the ward when they were allowed. We had cricket games in the halls or small ones in the rooms. Our wonderful medical team played along too, engaging in nerf gun fights and video games with Jake. They genuinely cared about him and his interests, keeping up with the latest gossip from reality TV shows and playing games together. These playful moments brought smiles to Jake's face and helped distract him from the challenges he was facing. It created a sense of camaraderie and friendship between him and the hospital staff, making the hospital feel like a more welcoming and friendly place. In those moments of joy and laughter, we forged lasting memories that reminded us of the resilience and spirit of our young fighter. Those small yet meaningful interactions were a testament to the power of human connection and the importance of finding moments of happiness even in the midst of difficult times.

BRAIN-FOG

Cancer-related cognitive impairment, commonly referred to as "cancer brain fog," "cancer fog," or "chemo brain" is a condition where some cancer patients experience changes in their cognitive abilities during and after treatment. These changes include difficulties with memory, concentration, and overall mental clarity, which can be frustrating and impact daily life. The exact causes of cancer brain fog are not fully understood, but it is reportedly influenced by various factors, including the cancer itself, treatments like chemotherapy, radiotherapy, and medications, as well as stress, fatigue, and emotional distress. The symptoms of cancer brain fog can vary in severity and may include memory problems, difficulty concentrating, slower processing speed, word finding difficulties, confusion, decreased attention span, and challenges with problem-solving.

Despite the challenges, there are strategies that can help manage the impact of cancer brain fog:

ENGAGING IN MINDFULNESS exercises and relaxation techniques can reduce stress and improve mental clarity.

REGULAR PHYSICAL ACTIVITY enhances cognitive function and reduces fatigue.

KEEPING THE BRAIN ACTIVE with puzzles, games, or learning new skills can help maintain cognitive abilities.

PRIORITIZING RESTFUL SLEEP is essential for mental clarity and overall well-being.

USING TOOLS like calendars, to-do lists, and reminders can assist in organization and planning daily tasks effectively.

A BALANCED DIET that includes brain-boosting foods can support cognitive function.

SEEKING EMOTIONAL SUPPORT and practical advice from healthcare providers, counsellors, or support groups is essential.

FOODS TO SUPPORT BRAIN FOG

CARBOHYDRATES: Complex carbohydrates, such as whole grains and sweet potatoes, provide a steady source of energy for the brain, helping to combat fatigue and support mental clarity.

EGGS: Eggs are rich in choline, an essential nutrient for memory and cognitive function. Including eggs in the diet can help support brain health.

BERRIES: Blueberries, strawberries, and other berries are packed with antioxidants that protect brain cells from oxidative stress, potentially enhancing cognitive function.

SALMON: Fatty fish, such as salmon, are excellent sources of omega-3 fatty acids, which play a crucial role in brain health and may aid in decreasing inflammation and supporting cognitive function.

LEAFY GREENS: Vegetables like spinach, kale, and broccoli contain nutrients like folate and vitamin K, which have been associated with improved cognitive function.

LIFESTYLE HABITS TO MANAGE BRAIN FOG

KEEP A CHECKLIST: Utilize checklists or task lists to stay organized and ensure important tasks are completed. This can help decrease feelings of overwhelm and increase productivity.

PUT THINGS IN THE SAME PLACE: Establish a consistent routine of putting items in designated places. This habit can lessen the frustration of misplacing things and enhance overall organization.

USE A CALENDAR: Maintain a calendar or planner to schedule appointments, events, and daily activities. This tool can help you keep track of your commitments and manage your time effectively.

DO ONE THING AT A TIME: Focusing on one task at a time can increase concentration and prevent mental fatigue. Avoid multitasking, when possible, to maintain mental clarity.

In conclusion, incorporating brain-supportive foods into the diet and adopting healthy lifestyle habits can be beneficial for managing cancer-related cognitive impairment. While these strategies may not completely eliminate brain fog, they can contribute to better cognitive function and overall well-being during and after cancer treatment. As always, it's essential to work closely with healthcare providers to address any concerns related to cancer brain fog and develop a comprehensive plan for support and management.

ADDITIONAL TIPS

SECOND-HAND SMOKE

Second-hand smoke, also known as passive smoke, involuntary smoke, environmental smoke, and environmental tobacco smoke, denotes smoke released from a person's cigar, cigarette, hookah, pipe, or any other tobacco-containing product. Involuntary exposure to second-hand smoke is known as second-hand smoking, which has been proven to be highly dangerous for non-smokers. The impact of smoking, especially second-hand smoke, on patients undergoing cancer treatment needs careful consideration. Research has established that exposure to second-hand smoke, even off clothes, hair, and indoor environments, can adversely affect stem cells in as little as 30 minutes. To protect the health of cancer patients, it is crucial to take measures to minimize exposure to second-hand smoke.

Hence, during cancer treatment, it is advisable to limit visits to family members' homes where smoking occurs. Instead, consider inviting them to your smoke-free environment. When extending invitations, kindly request that they shower and change into fresh clothes to minimize any lingering smoke residue. Most people will understand the importance of creating a smoke-free space for your well-being and will be supportive of such measures. By being proactive in addressing the issue of smoking, you can help safeguard your health and ensure a healthier environment during your cancer journey. It's vital to prioritise your well-being and communicate openly with family and friends about the impact of second-hand smoke on your health.

REFERENCES

Kim AS, Ko HJ, Kwon JH, et al. Exposure to secondhand smoke and risk of cancer in never smokers: a meta-analysis of epidemiologic studies. Int J Environ Res Public Health. 2018 Sep 11;15(9):1981. doi: 10.3390/ijerph15091981. PMID: 30208628; PMCID: PMC6164459.

American Association for Cancer Research. Secondhand smoke: impacting cancer survivors. Available at https://www.aacr.org/patients-caregivers/progress-against-cancer/secondhand-smoke-impacting-cancer-survivors/

Idris S, Baqays A, Isaac A, et al. The effect of second hand smoke in patients with squamous cell carcinoma of the head and neck. J Otolaryngol Head Neck Surg. 2019;48:33. https://doi.org/10.1186/s40463-019-0357-4

Rupnick MA, Panigrahy D, Zhang CY, et al. Adipose tissue mass can be regulated through the vasculature. Proc Natl Acad Sci U S A. 2002 Aug 6;99(16):10730-5. doi: 10.1073/pnas.162349799. Epub 2002 Jul 29. PMID: 12149466; PMCID: PMC125027.

HOUSEPLANTS DURING AND AFTER CANCER JOURNEY

Given below are some plants that you can have to create a favourable healing environment for your children during and after cancer treatment.

MADAGASCAR DRAGON TREE (or Dragon Tree) (Dracaena marginata): Renowned for its exceptional air-purifying qualities, dragon tree effectively eliminates harmful pollutants, such as benzene, trichloroethylene, and formaldehyde, from air, which have been linked to cancer and respiratory issues, making this plant a valuable addition to any indoor space.

SPIDER PLANT (Chlorophytum comosum): Another excellent air purifier, spider plant removes formaldehyde and xylene from air, which are commonly found in soft furnishings, solvents, and adhesives. The accumulation of these chemicals in home can lead to symptoms like dizziness, coughing, nausea, and headaches. Spider plant is an effective solution to combatting these indoor air contaminants.

COMMON IVY/ENGLISH IVY (Hedera helix): Known for its excellent filtration of cleaning products and airborne pollutants, such as mould, smoke, and dust, common ivy serves as a natural air purifier. Its ability to trap these harmful elements helps improve the overall air quality in home.

FLAMINGO FLOWER (Anthurium andreanum): An attractive and effective air-purifying plant, flamingo flower excels at removing formaldehyde, xylene, toluene, and ammonia from air, creating a healthier indoor environment.

CHINESE EVERGREEN (genus Aglaonema): Despite its modest size, Chinese evergreen boasts remarkable air-purifying capabilities. It can effectively remove pollutants like formaldehyde and benzene, while simultaneously increasing daytime oxygen levels, making it a valuable asset for improving indoor air quality.

PEACE LILY (genus Spathiphyllum): This plant has fantastic ability to filter a variety of toxins like benzene, acetone, formaldehyde, and trichloroethylene. Having it at home not just clears air but also promotes peace as reflected in its name.

By incorporating these air-purifying plants into your living space, you can create a healthier and more refreshing environment, free from harmful pollutants that could adversely affect your well-being.

REFERENCE:

Cameron R. HealthequalsFreedom. Indoor Plants and Cancer: Green Revolution – Health Equals Freedom. Available at https://www.healthequalsfreedom.com/environment/air/indoor-plants-and-cancer/

GROUNDING

Grounding, also known as earthing, is essential for children undergoing cancer treatment. This practice involves connecting with the Earth's surface to promote balance, relaxation, and overall well-being. Throughout cancer treatment, grounding helps children handle physical and emotional challenges they may encounter.

Grounding offers a myriad of benefits that contribute to children's healing journey:

STRESS REDUCTION: The cancer treatment process can be overwhelming for children, leading to increased stress and anxiety. Grounding techniques, such as walking barefoot on grass or soil, have been reported to reduce stress hormones and foster a sense of calm and relaxation.

IMPROVED SLEEP: Cancer treatments and hospital stays can disrupt children's sleep patterns. Grounding has been correlated with better sleep quality, enabling children to get the rest they need to support their healing process.

ENHANCED IMMUNE RESPONSE: Grounding has been linked to improved immune system function, which is vital for children undergoing cancer treatment to strengthen their defences against illness.

PAIN MANAGEMENT: Grounding has potential to help alleviate pain and discomfort related to cancer treatments, offering children a natural and non-invasive approach to managing pain.

EMOTIONAL SUPPORT: Engaging with nature through grounding can be emotionally comforting for children, providing them with a sense of connection, hope, and resilience throughout their cancer journey.

PRACTICING GROUNDING WITH CHILDREN

GROUNDING CAN BE PRACTICED WITH CHILDREN USING THE FOLLOWING

OUTDOOR PLAY: Encourage children to spend time outdoors, whether it's in the garden, a park, or a natural setting. Engaging in activities like running, playing, or simply sitting on the ground can facilitate grounding.

BAREFOOT WALKING: Encourage children to walk barefoot on natural surfaces, such as grass, sand, or soil. The direct contact with the Earth's surface promotes grounding and relaxation.

NATURE EXPLORATION: Take children on nature walks or hikes, enabling them to connect with the natural world and experience the calming and grounding effects of being in nature.

GARDENING: Involving children in gardening activities can be a grounding experience. Working with soil and plants fosters a sense of connection with the Earth and offers a therapeutic outlet.

MINDFUL PRACTICES: Teach children simple mindfulness exercises, such as deep breathing or guided meditations, to help them feel more grounded and centred.

INDOOR GROUNDING TOOLS: For times when outdoor activities are not possible, consider using indoor grounding tools, such as grounding mats or sheets, which are designed to connect with the Earth's energy.

As with any wellness practice, it's essential to consult with healthcare professionals and consider individual circumstances when introducing grounding to children during cancer treatment. Grounding can be a valuable complementary approach to support their overall well-being and provide them with additional tools for coping with the challenges they might face on their cancer journey.

REFERENCES

Oschman JL, Chevalier G, Brown R. The effects of grounding (earthing) on inflammation, the immune response, wound healing, and prevention and treatment of chronic inflammatory and autoimmune diseases. J Inflamm Res. 2015 Mar 24;8:83-96. doi: 10.2147/JIR.S69656. PMID: 25848315; PMCID: PMC4378297.

Menigoz W, Latz TT, Ely RA, et al. Integrative and lifestyle medicine strategies should include Earthing (grounding): Review of research evidence and clinical observations. Explore (NY). 2020 May-Jun;16(3):152-160. doi: 10.1016/j.explore.2019.10.005. Epub 2019 Nov 14. PMID: 31831261.

BUILDING RESILIENCE THROUGH PLAY

When it came to Jake's physical movements, we understood that it was vital for not only his physical health but also mental well-being. We considered ourselves fortunate to have a supportive environment where he could engage in physical play. Having his sisters to play with and his friends next door, along with living in a cul-de-sac, provided Jake with endless opportunities for fun and movement. When Jake felt up to it, they would ride their bikes around, build jumps, or have impromptu football matches. It was heart-warming to see them all active and having a blast together. If Jake started to feel tired, he had the option to sit outside and watch or come inside for a movie. On quieter days, we enjoyed activities like painting, playdough, or LEGO building competitions. These moments of play kept him moving, involved, and most importantly, distracted from the challenges of his treatment.

Some might wonder if letting him play so much was counterproductive, and that rest would be a better option. However, for us, seeing Jake's smiles and hearing his laughter was priceless. We trusted him to gauge his energy levels and slow down when needed. And, whenever he wanted to play, there was no way we would say no. We cherished every moment of fun, knowing that it could be the last time, and we were determined not to take those experiences away from him. It amazed his doctors too when he would excitedly tell them about his bike riding and other activities during appointments. They couldn't quite figure it out, especially when his blood levels were low. However, we knew that these moments of movement and joy were essential for Jake's spirit and determination.

Eventually, physical play became more than just a way to keep him active. It was an integral part of his healing journey, nurturing his mental resilience and happiness. It reminded us that life, even during cancer treatment, could still be filled with precious moments of joy and laughter. And as parents, we treasured those times as much as anything else.

During cancer treatment, the impact of exercise on gene expression and cell signalling pathways can offer several benefits for patients. Regarding gene expression, exercise can impact gene expression by increasing or decreasing the production of certain proteins. For example, exercise can upregulate genes responsible for antioxidant defence and energy metabolism, while downregulate genes related to inflammation. Regarding cell signalling pathways, exercise can activate various cell signalling pathways, which can trigger cascades of molecular events that affect gene expression and cellular function. These pathways play a role in processes like muscle adaptation, repair, and growth.

HERE'S HOW THESE PROCESSES CAN BE ADVANTAGEOUS

Enhanced Antioxidant Defence: The upregulation of genes involved in antioxidant defence can be mainly beneficial for cancer patients. Cancer treatments, such as chemotherapy and radiotherapy, generate oxidative stress that can damage healthy cells. Therefore, increased antioxidant activity may help mitigate some of this damage, reducing treatment-related side effects and supporting overall well-being.

IMPROVED ENERGY METABOLISM: Upregulating genes related to energy metabolism can support patients during cancer treatment, as they often experience fatigue and reduced energy levels. Enhanced energy metabolism may provide patients with increased stamina and help them manage daily activities better, enhancing their quality of life.

REDUCED INFLAMMATION: Downregulating inflammation-related genes can benefit cancer patients, as chronic inflammation is associated with disease progression and treatment side effects. By limiting inflammation, exercise may contribute to a supplementary favourable treatment response and alleviate some treatment-related symptoms.

MUSCLE ADAPTATION AND REPAIR: Activation of cell signalling pathways through exercise supports muscle adaptation and repair. Cancer treatment can result in muscle wasting and weakness, making it challenging for patients to sustain their physical strength. Hence, regular exercise can help combat muscle loss, improving functional capacity and overall physical resilience.

IMMUNE FUNCTION SUPPORT: Exercise influences the immune system positively. For cancer patients, a well-functioning immune system is vital for combatting the disease and minimizing the risk of infections, which can be more challenging to handle during treatment.

PSYCHOLOGICAL WELL-BEING: The positive effects of exercise on gene expression and cell signalling pathways can also extend to mental health. Engaging in physical activity can lower stress, anxiety, and depression, offering much-needed emotional support for patients dealing with the emotional toll of cancer treatment.

MEDIATING TREATMENT Side Effects: Exercise can mitigate the side effects of cancer treatments. By boosting antioxidant defence and decreasing inflammation, patients may experience fewer treatment-related complications, allowing them to better tolerate therapy and uphold their treatment schedule.

ENHANCED TREATMENT EFFICACY: While exercise is not a replacement for cancer treatment, its potential impact on gene expression and cell signalling pathways may complement therapy. By improving overall health and well-being, exercise may enhance the body's ability to respond to treatment and support the body's natural defences against cancer cells.

Of note, exercise during cancer treatment should be tailored to individual circumstances, considering the patient's overall health, treatment regimen, and energy levels. In addition, healthcare team should always be consulted before starting an exercise program to ensure its safety and appropriateness for patient-specific situation.

As I close this book, I find myself overwhelmed with emotions. This journey through childhood cancer treatment has been challenging, yet filled with moments of hope and resilience.

Through sharing my experiences and those of children like Jake, I hope that this book can provide comfort and support to other families facing similar battles.

From the very beginning, I knew that childhood cancer treatment would be tough, but I never anticipated the rollercoaster of emotions that we would endure. The diagnosis hit us like a wrecking ball, and I felt lost and scared. Nevertheless, in the midst of it all, we found strength in each other and the unwavering support of our healthcare team. Throughout Jake's treatment, we faced numerous hurdles and tough decisions, especially when it came to using an NG tube to ensure he received proper nutrition and medication. It was a challenging journey, and I often questioned if we were doing the right thing. However, Jake's resilience and courage inspired us to keep pushing forward.

One of the most unexpected revelations came when we noticed Jake's self-perception changing because of the presence of the NG tube. When we accidentally removed it during playtime, we were prepared for tears and breakdowns. However, something remarkable happened. Jake seemed more liberated and happier without it. It made me realise the emotional impact the tube had on him, and we made the decision to keep it out as he neared the end of his treatment. Watching him embrace life with newfound joy was incredibly heart-warming.

Through this journey, I learned the value of celebrating even the smallest victories. Each milestone, whether it was completing a round of treatment or trying a new food, was cause for celebration. I also learned the importance of staying positive and providing unwavering support for Jake, his sisters, and our entire family. As we reached the end of Jake's treatment, I couldn't help but feel a mix of emotions: relief, gratitude, and hope filled my heart. Though the road was tough, it brought us closer as a family and reminded us of the strength we have within us.

To all the families out there facing childhood cancer, know that you are not alone. There is a whole community of parents, caregivers, and healthcare professionals who stand beside you. Embrace the journey with hope, love, and resilience. Even on the darkest days, remember that there is light at the end of the tunnel. As I close this chapter of our lives, I am filled with gratitude for the support we received, the lessons we learned, and the precious moments we shared. To every child who has battled cancer, you are true warriors, and your strength continues to inspire others. Together, let us look towards a future filled with hope, healing, and a world where childhood cancer is no more.

Thank you from the depths of my heart for being a part of this journey with me. Your presence and support have meant the world to me. I hope this book has offered comfort and inspiration to those facing childhood cancer challenges. Sharing our experiences and insights has been a profound experience, and knowing that we are not alone in this battle has brought immense strength. Let us continue to stand together with hope for a brighter future where childhood cancer is conquered.

With heartfelt gratitude,

GLOSSARY

AMINO ACIDS: Small molecules that are the building blocks of proteins (proteins serve as the structural support inside the cell and perform many vital chemical reactions).

ANTIOXIDANT: A substance that protects the body against the effects of free radicals, toxins, and pollution.

ASPIRATION: Accidental inhalation of any foreign object or substance into your airway.

BETA-CRYPTOXANTHIN/CRYPTOXANTHIN: A strong antioxidant with a particular effect on reducing the risk of certain cancers.

BRAIN FOG: A condition where some cancer patients experience changes in their cognitive abilities during and after treatment.

CALCIUM: Helps maintain healthy, strong, and dense teeth and bones. Inadequate calcium intake may lead to weak bones as the body takes calcium from them to meet its needs.

ELECTROLYTES: Minerals that carry an electrical charge. Electrolytes support cell function, energy production, hydration, and muscle contractions, including the heartbeat.

ENTERAL FEEDING: Method of feeding where a specific amount of liquid nutrition is delivered directly into the stomach or small intestines through a feeding tube at set intervals throughout the day.

ENTERAL NUTRITION: Enteral feeding provided in the hospital setting.

HOME ENTERAL NUTRITION: Enteral feeding provided outside the hospital setting, at home mostly.

HYPERPHAGIA (polyphagia): A feeling of extreme, insatiable hunger, which could occur in patients undergoing cancer treatment.

INSULIN: A hormone produced by the pancreas that regulates blood sugar levels.

IRON: A mineral needed for growth and development. The body uses iron to make haemoglobin, a protein in red blood cells that carries oxygen throughout the body.

LUTEIN: Carotenes, yellow / red / orange pigments found in food, a variety of plants, and egg yolk. Lutein is a powerful antioxidant that defends your body against unstable molecules.

MAGNESIUM: A nutrient that the body needs to be healthy. It helps regulate the body, including muscle and nerve function, blood sugar levels, blood pressure, and the production of protein for the bones and DNA.

NASOGASTRIC TUBE: A medical device inserted through the nose and down the throat into the stomach to deliver nutrition, fluids, or medications to individuals who cannot consume these substances orally.

OMEGA-3: Types of polyunsaturated fat that are vital for normal body functions. They provide a range of health benefits and protect against various diseases.

PECTIN: A soluble fibre found in citrus fruits and apples. It aids in reducing bad cholesterol levels.

POLYPHENOL: Plant chemicals that include bioflavonoids, phenols, quercetin, and tannins. Polyphenols help manage blood pressure, keep blood vessels healthy and flexible, promote good circulation, and reduce chronic inflammation.

POTASSIUM: A mineral that your body needs to function properly. It aids in nerve function and muscle contraction, helps regulate your heartbeat, and facilitates the movement of nutrients into cells and waste products out of cells.

PREBIOTICS: Compounds found in many foods that stimulate the growth of beneficial bacteria in the intestines.

PROBIOTICS: Friendly gut bacteria that boost the immune system.

RECOMMENDED DIETARY INTAKE (RDI): The average daily dietary intake level that is sufficient to meet nutrient requirements.

SECOND-HAND SMOKE: Smoke released from a person's cigar, cigarette, hookah, pipe, or any other tobacco-containing product.

TOTAL PARENTERAL NUTRITION: A specialized medical treatment in which essential nutrients, including carbohydrates, proteins, fats, vitamins, and minerals, are delivered directly into a child's bloodstream through an intravenous (IV) line.

VITAMIN B: A group of vitamins that are well-known for helping the body unlock the energy it needs to function well. They are also linked to improving stress levels.

VITAMIN C: An essential nutrient found in many fruits and vegetables. The body needs vitamin C to form and maintain bones, blood vessels, and skin.

VITAMIN D: The body requires a small amount to stay healthy and function properly. Vitamin D helps the body use calcium and phosphorus to build strong bones and teeth.

VITAMIN E: An antioxidant that may help repair damaged cells against free radicals.

VITAMIN E: Helps the nerves and muscles work well, prevents blood clots, and boosts the immune system.

ZINC: Provides benefits such as aiding the immune system and metabolism function. It is also important for wound healing.

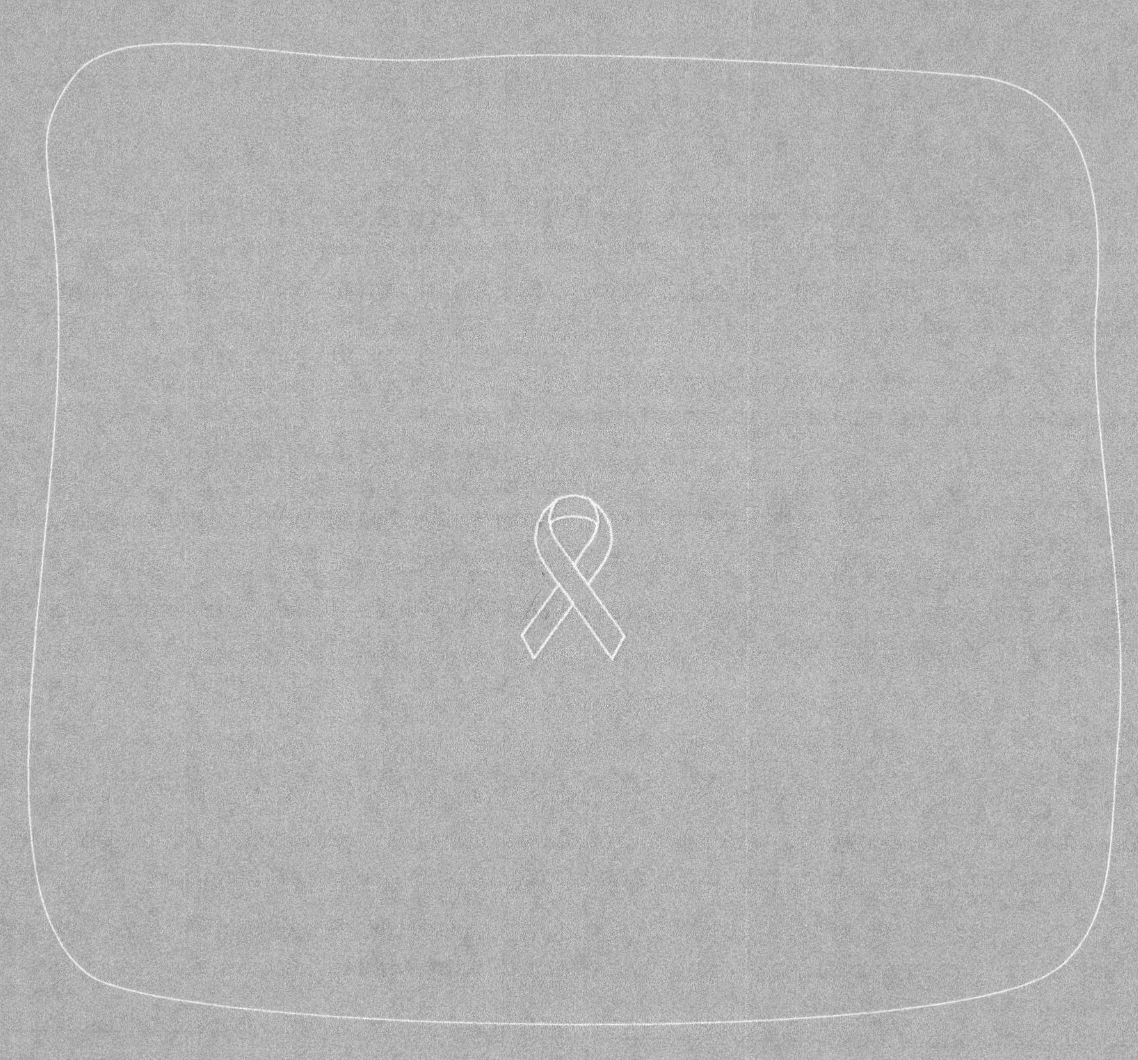

The information provided in this book is intended for general purposes only. While every effort has been made to ensure the accuracy of the contents, it should not be treated as a substitute for qualified medical advice. Always consult a qualified medical practitioner. Neither the author nor the publisher can be held responsible for any loss or claim arising from the use or misuse of the suggestions provided or the failure to seek appropriate advice.

Maintaining a good baseline of health and well-being during and after cancer treatment depends on adopting a healthy diet. Recent research indicates a correlation among diet, weight control, regular exercise, and improved survival rates. These factors have also been established contribute to decreased cancer recurrence in those in remission and may even aid in disease prevention.